Non-Fee-for-Service Revenue Cycle Management

MANAGING PATIENT SERVICE AND CLINICAL PERFORMANCE TO MAXIMIZE HEALTHCARE PRACTICE PROFIT

RONALD B. STERLING, CPA, MBA

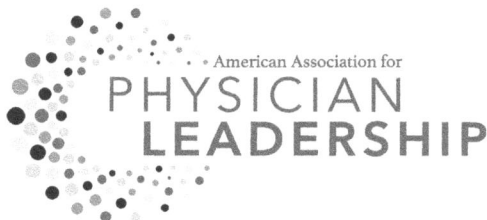

American Association for
PHYSICIAN
LEADERSHIP

Copyedited, typeset, indexed, and printed in the United States of America

PUBLISHER
Nancy Collins

EDITORIAL ASSISTANT
Jennifer Weiss

DESIGN & LAYOUT
Carter Publishing Studio

COPYEDITOR
Pat George

TABLE OF CONTENTS

Presents the key issues that practices/HCOs need to address to succeed in the non-FFS environment.

Provides strategic context to the differences between the FFS and non-FFS arrangements.

Examines the impact of non-FFS models on physician compensation and presents considerations and strategies to adjust physician compensation to address changes in revenue producing activities as well as maximize physician contributions to patient care and practice/HCO success.

Reviews the key features of FFS focused PMS tools and how PMS features can be repurposed to support the more varied and complex aspects of non-FFS billing and payments.

Examines how CEHRT features can be used to support and track non-FFS oriented patient care and services. Includes sections on remote patient monitoring, telemedicine and patient portals.

Focuses on the use of treatment plans to reinforce and document patient care and practice/HCO due diligence. Reviews the importance and significance of treatment order status and review features.

Assesses the significance of clinical call centers for non-FFS arrangements as well as transition issues from current patient service strategies.

CHAPTERS 7–12:

A chapter is included for each non-FFS model to explain how the model operates and the performance and payment posting challenges of each situation. Each chapter includes sections on managerial accounting and policy issues as well as patient service, practice management system, electronic health record, and reporting considerations.

Non-FFS situations require close attention to monitoring clinical performance and patient services. This chapter includes monitoring strategies for key items to assure meeting your performance and service requirements.

Concludes with strategic context for your continuing efforts.

ABOUT THE AUTHOR

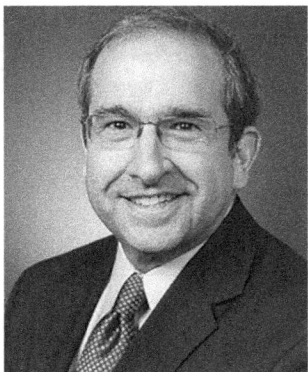

Ronald B. Sterling, CPA, MBA, president of Sterling Solutions, Ltd. (www.sterling-solutions.com), is a nationally recognized thought leader on healthcare information technology. He has guided a wide array of healthcare organizations to capitalize on technology to improve patient service, control costs and maximize revenue.

A HIMSS Book of the Year winning author, Ron has written eight books on healthcare IT, including *Keys to EHR Success,* published by Greenbranch Publishing. He has authored hundreds of articles on healthcare information technology for dozens of publications including *Medscape.* He also serves on the Medscape Business of Medicine Advisory Board.

Ron frequently speaks on healthcare technology to a variety of provider and industry groups. His presentations include:
- Medicare Quality Payment Program
- Non-Fee-for-Service Revenue Cycle Management and Analytics
- Physician Compensation Under Non-Fee for Service Arrangements
- Clinical End of Day—Protecting Patient Service and Patient Records
- HIPAA Privacy and Security.

Ron earned a B.S. in Information Systems from the University of Maryland and an MBA in International Business from George Washington University. He is a member of the AICPA and Maryland Association of CPAs.

Contact Information:
Ron Sterling, CPA, MBA
Sterling Solutions, Ltd.
Email: rbsterling@sterling-solutions.com
Phone: (301) 681-4247

ACKNOWLEDGMENTS

In my conversations with Nancy Collins of Greenbranch Publishing on a variety of healthcare industry issues and healthcare information technology, she often says "Why don't you write another book?" So, I did.

Nancy was the publisher of *Keys to EHR Success,* a HIMSS Book of the Year. She has moved mountains of paper to get this book in your hands because she believes that you need this information now. Indeed, you should start working on developing a plan to deal with the billing, management, and analytic issues of non-fee for service arrangements now . . . in 2017.

I appreciate the opportunity to work with Nancy again.

I also want to thank Beth Matosko for keeping things running at Sterling Solutions for over 20 years. She has been helpful and supportive in getting things done.

I would have never made it to step one in this process without the support of my wife, Janis. She has been incredible through the ups and downs of the business cycle and is the key to my personal life. She has been my indispensable partner in raising our four kids to become incredible adults.

This book is dedicated to my parents, Hannah and Kenneth Sterling, who passed away within five weeks of each other in 2015. They had the inspiring life stories that earned the Greatest Generation its name. From challenging childhoods through the Depression to World War II (my Dad served in the Army and my Mom worked for the Army), they moved forward to build a better life for themselves and their family. My parents (and their generation) were resilient, creative, productive, and inspirational. I will lovingly remember their hard work and unconditional commitment to their family and country.

Thank you,

RON STERLING

GLOSSARY

ACI—Advancing Care Information

ACO—Accountable Care Organization

CDS—Clinical Decision Support

CEHRT—Certified Electronic Health Record Technology

EOC—Episode of Care

FFS—Fee for Service

HCO—Healthcare Organization

MIPS—Merit-Based Incentive Payment System

Non-FFS—Non-Fee for Service

PMS—Practice Management System

RPM—Remote Patient Monitoring

RPMS—Remote Patient Monitoring System

Introduction

Non-fee for service (non-FFS) revenue cycle management is a continuous process that affects your clinical and administrative strategies and tactics. It begins before you see the first patient, with analysis of what the practice/healthcare organization (HCO) needs to succeed, as well as a feasibility analysis of how to meet the standards of a non-FFS arrangement.

The practice/HCO proceeds to develop accommodations for the specific plan in the practice management system (PMS)/certified electronic health record technology (CEHRT), operations, clinical services and other practice/HCO functions. Once patients are seen, the practice/HCO continuously monitors patient and practice activities to ensure that the non-FFS requirements are met and the revenue earned. Then the next non-FFS arrangement may present a completely different set of challenges and issues.

As the healthcare system migrates from the FFS model to a variety of non-FFS payment systems, a wide range of processes, strategies, and tools designed for FFS could inhibit your ability to analyze your clinical and/or financial performance. From managing services that generate revenue, to billing, to tracking clinical and business performance, the non-FFS models present resource, patient service, billing, and reporting challenges.

Non-FFS revenue cycle management arrangements do not exist in a vacuum or represent an exclusive arrangement with a payer or any other sponsoring organizations. Indeed, you may continue to have a FFS arrangement with a payer that includes a non-FFS based shared savings component. On the other hand, a specialist may see an FFS arrangement replaced with a non-FFS case or episode of care payment.

The challenge of managing non-FFS arrangements exceeds the typical requirements to manage your FFS-based relationships. To date, practices/HCOs may have a couple of non-FFS arrangements that do not represent a substantive percentage of their patient or revenue base. For example, when calculating profitability, many practices/HCOs combine non-FFS revenue in a pool that offsets operational costs.

However, more and more non-FFS arrangements will affect clinical responsibilities and require a more precise analysis for managing the practice, determining profitability, and compensating physicians. For example, the Medicare Advanced Alternative Payment Model (APM) incentivizes providers and groups to have 50% of Medicare patients or 75% of Medicare revenue under non-FFS arrangements under an Advanced APM by 2021.

Non-FFS arrangements can dramatically differ in performance requirements, terms, and patient focus. The diversity and complexity of these arrangements require a new look at how practices/HCOs manage and analyze their clinical operations, patient relationships, and financial performance. In some cases, a new set of tactics and monitoring strategies will be needed to meet patient service and payer requirements.

With that in mind, the key questions facing your organization are:

What are the clinical and operational requirements to earn the non-FFS revenue?

Depending on the goals and objectives of the payer, the non-FFS arrangement could include general goals or specific activities needed to succeed. Some of these requirements may be a natural byproduct of your current FFS procedures and others may require a more expansive view of patient service and management. For example, the non-FFS strategy may rely on more active patient engagement outside of the office, which may not be a current FFS tactic.

Unfortunately, each non-FFS arrangement could have different measures, requirements, and payment triggers. The challenge is to successfully meet individual non-FFS arrangements without sacrificing practice/HCO efficiency and patient relationships.

How will the practice/HCO track clinical performance and patient service that could impact non-FFS revenue?

Once the practice/HCO understands the patient service and operational requirements, it should assess the readiness of its staff, policies, procedures, and tools to accommodate the non-FFS program. The practice/HCO may repurpose PMS/CEHRT tools to facilitate treating patients within the non-FFS standards as well as monitor how well the practice/HCO meets the non-FFS standards. In so doing, the practice/HCO will ensure that performance incentives are earned. In other situations, the practice/HCO will have the information needed to challenge the non-FFS sponsor in the event of a discrepancy between the practice/HCO results and the sponsor's "scorecard."

What costs are incurred in producing the non-FFS revenue?

The practice/HCO could be facing new expenses to meet the non-FFS program requirements or incur the costs of new strategies dictated by the non-FFS program. For example, the non-FFS program may require electronic reporting that is charged separately by your PMS/CEHRT vendor. In some cases, the costs of non-FFS efforts may be shared by several different arrangements. For example, the practice/HCO may need to set up a clinical call center that would be used to fulfill requirements for several non-FFS relationships.

The non-FFS program costs affect the physician compensation strategy for non-FFS revenues. For example, the practice/HCO may set up a cost center for the call center and charge the costs to the non-FFS program before calculating physician distributions.

The estimated costs of supporting the non-FFS program may be considered in your negotiations with the non-FFS sponsor. For example, the practice/HCO may be able to get an advance payment to fund the new patient service setups required by the non-FFS program.

How will the practice/HCO verify that the non-FFS payment is correct?

Each non-FFS arrangement will have a payment calculation method and payment cycle. The practice/HCO should maintain sufficient information to verify the calculation and payment amount. For example, the practice/HCO may have reports to verify the number of patients under a capitation plan or the quality measure used to calculate the non-FFS payment.

How will non-FFS revenue be credited to physicians in calculating their compensation?

Applying the non-FFS revenue in the same way that FFS revenue is applied may be difficult. Non-FFS revenue is not necessarily a function of physician-billed services and cannot necessarily be directly attributed to a doctor. For example, a lump-sum performance incentive may be paid based on practice/HCO performance. The practice/HCO will need to develop internal measurements and policies to allocate non-FFS receipts to physicians. For example, the practice/HCO may allocate non-FFS payments by number of patients managed by the doctor.

What are the analytical tools needed to evaluate the financial performance of the non-FFS arrangement?

The various performance requirements and measurements associated with a non-FFS plan must be worked into your PMS/CEHRT strategy. For example, the practice/HCO may:

- Set up a patient class to track the number of patients served by a health coach;
- Establish a charge code to flag patients who attend a free weight counseling class as part of the non-FFS treatment program; or
- Use a monthly charge code to indicate use of remote patient monitoring for a patient.

The practice/HCO must track non-FFS requirements as well as generate reports and analyses to monitor non-FFS performance through PMS/CEHRT reports, worklists, and other tools.

Non-Fee for Service Revenue Cycle Management helps you plan approaches that will fulfill non-FFS obligations as well as capitalize on the financial opportunities of non-FFS arrangements.

Chapter 1, Why Non-FFS Is a Challenge, further explores the underlying issues and tests facing your practice/HCO in a more diversified and complicated patient service and operational environment.

Chapter 2, Physician Compensation, examines the effect of non-FFS revenue streams and offers several strategies to equitably distribute revenue to physicians and other providers.

Chapters 3–6 cover the wide range of tools of the trade that you need to succeed in the non-FFS based environment. The chapters cover the essential considerations, strategies, and tactics needed to support the non-FFS healthcare environment as follows:

- **Practice Management Systems (Chapter 3)**
- **Electronic Health Records (Chapter 4)**
- **Orders (Chapter 5)**
- **Clinical Call Center (Chapter 6)**

Chapters 7–12 examine the various issues associated with the key non-FFS models that the practice/HCO will be dealing with.

- **MIPS Adjustments (Chapter 7)**
- **Performance and Quality Incentives (Chapter 8)**
- **Care Management (Chapter 9)**
- **Shared Savings (Chapter 10)**
- **Episode of Care (Chapter 11)**
- **Capitation Payments (Chapter 12)**

Chapter 13, Monitoring Operations and Patient Information, discusses the day-to-day activities needed to maintain the integrity of your PMS/CEHRT information to support your non-FFS obligations and maintain the integrity of the patient record.

Chapter 14, Go-Forward Strategy, summarizes the strategy you need to succeed with your ever-growing revenue driven by non-FFS arrangements.

CHAPTER 1

Why Non-FFS Is a Challenge

FFS arrangements are relatively straightforward. For participation with a payer, the practice/HCO signs an agreement that includes a fee schedule. After clinical reviews and other details, the practice can provide services to patients and submit claims under a negotiated fee schedule. If the practice/HCO is not a participating provider, the organization serves the patient, submits claims, and awaits payment based on what the payer determines is the appropriate compensation for the service. The billable service is a distinct activity that has a precise start and stop. Complicating FFS arrangements are surgical procedures that include a global period.

Non-FFS arrangements typically include a range of obligations and measures that require sustained excellence for multiple patients over a month, several months, or even a year to earn revenue. The practice/HCO may have to perform several activities around patient encounters or even in place of patient encounters. Therefore, the non-FFS onboarding process requires more analysis to uncover important adjustments to the clinical and administrative operations before the practice/HCO is ready to take on patients. For example, the non-FFS program may require use of designated labs and testing groups, or require the practice/HCO to provide enhanced therapy services using a specific protocol. After the patients are being served, the practice/HCO may have to continuously monitor clinical operations to sustain patient services at the non-FFS required performance level.

Many practices/HCOs will be struggling with these non-FFS driven patient service and care models. Other practices/HCOs may have innovative tools, techniques, and strategies to succeed with the non-FFS arrangements. Such accomplishments may become a competitive advantage in working with the payer as well as serving patients. For example, if few practices are meeting the non-FFS requirements, your practice/HCO may be a preferred provider.

Success with non-FFS arrangements depends on the ability of providers and staff to efficiently serve and monitor patients. In some cases, the practice/HCO is completely responsible for meeting the goals of the non-FFS plan. For example, the practice/HCO may provide a full range of services to address an injury and rehabilitate the patient. In other non-FFS programs, the non-FFS payer may specify strategy and performance measures for the practice/HCO to earn bonuses and incentives. For example, a cardiology practice may receive a performance incentive based on seeing referred patients within two weeks after a primary care referral.

Non-FFS models require a more coordinated approach to serving and managing patients. One of the key objectives of many non-FFS models is to improve patient adherence to care plans and healthier lifestyles to improve or maintain patient wellness. This coordinated approach requires a new look at the tactics and strategies used to treat patients as well as more active and frequent engagement with the patient on care issues.

CHAPTER 2

Physician Compensation

U nder FFS, many physicians are paid based on a percentage of the billings or collections as well as a formula tied to Relative Value Units (RVUs). These compensation arrangements were designed for targeted services that produce a (mostly) reliable reimbursement from the payer. Outside of the patient not being covered or the service not being properly authorized, the claim would be paid. For the most part, each patient encounter stood on its own and was not subject to at-risk reimbursement across an entire body of patients.

Non-FFS revenue poses physician compensation dilemmas because receipt of payments may be partially or tangentially connected to physician specific services. For example,

- A case manager may assure adherence to a therapy program managed by occupation and physical therapists.
- The practice may receive a performance payment attached to more effective management of patients by staff and mid-level providers.

A successful patient service strategy to ensure and monitor adherence to physician recommendations for health as well as therapy may result in fewer office visits offset by incentive payments for saving money or monitoring patients.

Non-FFS payments may involve significant new non-physician expenses. For example,

- The practice/HCO may maintain a call center staffed with mid-level providers and nurses that generate shared savings or other non-FFS revenues.
- A fee per patient per month may include remote patient management tools that cost the practice/HCO a monthly fee. The out-of-pocket cost could vary by the types and number of monitoring tools used by each patient.

- Physicians who personally manage every patient service may transition to a more collaborative patient service strategy utilizing nurses for patient outreach and education as well as PAs for treating patients under the supervision of the doctor to meet productivity and patient service requirements.
- Non-FFS strategies may require additional clinical staff and investments in training on patient service strategies that may be new to the practice/HCO. In some cases, the tactics may be specific to the non-FFS plan.

Non-FFS revenue may be based on additional work and effort outside of the FFS-based services provided by the same practice. For example, the practice may be paid on an FFS basis for a select group of CPT® codes as well as receive payments not connected to any service codes for success with patients and cost reduction.

In theory, you could experience a decrease in physician reimbursement due to lower level of services enabled by the incentivized non-FFS arrangement. For example, your practice may replace monthly physician visits with bi-weekly telemedicine encounters with a nurse or PA while the patient is seen by the doctor based on the telemedicine strategy. The implications of these changes are substantial:

- Physicians may need a larger base of patients to keep the appointment book filled and office busy. For example, if a problem typically requires a weekly patient visit for wound care, the practice may be able to use telemedicine and other patient management techniques to replace office visits. In that way, the patient is served at less cost while having more contact with the practice/HCO. From an efficiency perspective, these strategies will require fewer physician services but additional practice/HCO staff efforts per patient. Doctors who want to maintain their CPT® services revenue level must balance their patient service monitoring efforts with a larger panel of patients to yield the same level of office visits, and procedures.
- Although doctors may benefit from non-FFS profits from other practice/HCO activities, they will need to spend time establishing clinical protocols for staff and mid-level providers as well as monitoring clinical and call center activities. For example, clinical staff may follow up with patients on the status of their health problem and guide patients using

the treatment plan defined by the doctor. Some practices/HCOs may assign doctors to monitor the call center.

- Non-physician resources present an additional cost that must be accommodated and budgeted into non-FFS payments. For example, the practice/HCO may set up cost centers to be allocated to non-FFS revenue before allocating the remaining revenue to physicians.

Considering the variety of differences between the non-FFS arrangements and the FFS business model, practices/HCOs need to develop physician compensation strategies that reflect the costs and changes in patient service patterns driven by non-FFS reimbursement. The key questions include:

How will costs be allocated to non-FFS revenue?

The practice/HCO may have additional costs associated with general strategy as well as specific costs to fulfill a non-FFS contract. For example, a non-FFS contract may require new patient education materials or 24/7 monitoring of incoming patient information. The practice/HCO needs to track costs and develop a mechanism to allocate the costs to non-FFS arrangements and any other expenses such as out-of-pocket testing to determine the revenue available for physician compensation.

How should adjustments to fees be credited to physicians?

Medicare Merit-based Incentive Payment System (MIPS) is an example of how adjustments are made to the fees paid to the practice. In other situations, a non-FFS arrangement may be based on a reduced-fee schedule for CPT® services supplemented by non-FFS payments for patient service and/or performance.

> *TIP*: Reduced fees may also be tracked to verify the realization of the non-FFS arrangement.

Depending on the situation, practices/HCOs may want to segregate non-FFS-driven payment adjustments that are affected by non-FFS arrangements and allocate the adjustments through another mechanism. For example, the adjustments could be used to offset additional costs for the non-FFS program and the remaining monies allocated to physicians based on charges, patient base, and/or contribution to earning the non-FFS revenue. A doctor may invest a lot of time guiding patient interventions that decrease office visits, but generate substantial shared savings payments.

When developing the physician compensation strategy, the practice/HCO needs to consider the performance baseline for all providers. If a physician does not support the performance requirements and is reimbursed at a lower level, the practice/HCO must decide how potential revenue loses are handled. For example, consider the MIPS adjustment example:

> One provider does nothing and is assigned a negative 4% adjustment and another provider does everything and gets a positive 4% adjustment plus part of the $500M bonus pool in 2019. The lower MIPS scored doctor would receive $96 for a $100 claim and the higher MIPS performing provider would receive $114 ($4 for the MIPS adjustment and $10 for an outstanding MIPS score.)

> If the doctors are paid 50% of their receipts, then the lower-performing provider will be contributing $2 less (50% of the $4 negative adjustment to the $100 claim) to practice expenses while the higher MIPS scorer would be contributing $9 more to practice expenses than the lower-performing provider (50% of the $18 difference between the $96 and $114 remittances).

Such differences could be manifested in many ways among and within non-FFS arrangements. For example, doctors could use different treatment plans under case management or doctors could differ regarding techniques and commitment to saving expenses under a shared savings arrangement.

To equitably distribute money among clinicians, the practice/HCO may need to track internal performance by provider and use non-FFS support as a factor in physician and clinician compensation. For example, the practice/HCO may compare the average episode of care cost among doctors in the practice as well as national cost averages. The key policy issues to consider follow.

Should non-FFS payments be adjusted before crediting receipts to physicians?

The practice/HCO may incur costs to support the non-FFS arrangement. For example, out-of-pocket costs such as remote patient monitoring services could be directly costed to the patient and payer plan. Similarly, you may establish a set price for clinical call center support or allocate a per-call/contact charge based on the staff level (i.e., nurse, or PA) servicing the patient.

How will physicians be credited with non-FFS revenue generation not directly attributed to the physician?

Non-FFS success is based on effective clinical care as well as practice/HCO help and guidance for patients. Numerous measures are available to determine success, including quality measures, and internal performance measures that help the practice/HCO manage patient service and care. For example, a practice may require an active treatment plan for all current patients.

Strategies to support these efforts must be based on physician involvement. Clinical consideration and patient wellness must be considered when establishing the non-FFS strategy and tactics, as well as continuing efforts to monitor performance and patient care. Practices/HCOs will need to determine how to recognize physician efforts and contributions to non-FFS programs outside of the office visit. For example, physician compensation may include an allocation for managing clinical standards or an innovative care strategy for a non-FFS program.

How will payments be credited to individual physicians?

After the practice/HCO develops its strategy for allocating costs and the timing of revenue recognition, a plan for allocating revenue to physicians can be created. The challenge is that non-FFS revenue will represent an increasing portion of revenues and any mistakes in allocations would be problematic. For example, a simplistic non-FFS revenue allocation may overstate physician revenue and lead to cash shortages and underpaying the people who are dedicated to supporting the non-FFS arrangement. Indeed, the lack of an organized approach to non-FFS physician income could undermine the ability of the practice to meet non-FFS performance and patient service requirements that drive revenue and profits.

The practice should have a general structure to address each non-FFS type as well as plan-specific adjustments for the nuances of a plan. For example, the scope of covered services and patient management tasks may vary.

The practice should have a mechanism for each plan for each period to calculate the distribution to the physicians as follows:

Determine revenue earned from the non-FFS plan. The specifics of the non-FFS plan will drive the recognition of revenue. The payment should be evaluated for the relevant period. Payments in advance should be evaluated after the close of the next month, while payments for the prior month would be evaluated for activity in the month just ended.

The allocation of revenue may span periods and will require close attention to cash flow. For example, an episode of care fee may have to be allocated over a period of several months to ensure that funds are available for follow-up care and patient service. Similarly, reserving portions of capitation payments for future services may be a reasonable approach to address a growing capitation base.

> *CAUTION*: Holding cash for future expenses could prove a problem for cash basis practices/HCOs at the end of a year. For example, cash being held for future services may result in taxable income to owners of a cash based practice/HCO.

In other instances, the practice/HCO needs to avoid a cash crunch. For example, failing to allocate out-of-pocket expenses to an incentive payment could leave no money to pay for remote patient monitoring services.

Subtract non-FFS costs to the plan for the period. The practice/HCO may have non-physician costs that are mission critical for the non-FFS situation. For example, the costs of the call center could be allocated through a per-patient charge for each non-FFS plan or derived from the services for patients under the plan. The non-FFS costs could include hard costs such as remote patient monitoring charges or lab tests.

Subtract support and management costs needed to fulfill the non-FFS requirements. The practice/HCO may have other costs that are allocated to the non-FFS plans through an allocation. For example, the practice/HCO may have expenses for patient education or an electronic interface with a patient portal that is required by the non-FFS plan. Such costs may be required for a specific plan or may be shared by several plans.

Distribute remaining revenue. The remaining revenue can be distributed to the physicians per practice/HMO rules. For example,

- Revenue could be distributed to physicians based on their quality and clinical performance measures. In other cases, revenue distributions could be based on the number of doctor's patients under the non-FFS plan.

- Physicians may be able to block patients from the non-FFS plan or due to the nature of the plan, the physician may not see patients from a plan. In these cases, physicians who do not serve patients may not receive money from the plan.
- A physician with low performance-measure scores used by the payer to calculate a non-FFS incentive may receive a smaller portion of the payment. Indeed, the practice/HCO may establish a distribution formula that includes credit for meeting the plan objectives and the number of plan patients served.

> *ALERT*: The practice/HCO has a vested interest in succeeding with all doctors. Therefore, the practice/HCO should monitor the payer performance measures at the provider level.

> *TIP*: The practice may want to include the physician's performance in maintaining records per monitoring operations (See Chapter 13).

The net amount paid to the physician would be depend on how the practice/HCO allocates expenses. For example, some organizations pay a percentage of physician-attributed revenue less an overhead rate and physician benefits while others directly allocate expenses to each physician. Some practices/HCO directly charge physicians for their nursing staff and mid-level assistants.

These non-FFS tactics are much more complicated than the FFS-based physician compensation models. Indeed, practices have been dealing with a low level of non-FFS arrangements for many years. However, the success or failure of these low-volume arrangements were not substantive compared to FFS volume. The move to non-FFS models and higher at-risk arrangements requires a new look at compensation and incentivizing performance.

The changing healthcare business models are increasing the importance of non-FFS business. Failure to meet non-FFS requirements could have a substantial effect on financial performance. Failure can result in penalties or lost opportunities to earn incentive and performance payments. To maximize revenue and allocate non-FFS revenues that are fair to the practice/HCO and providers requires a new look at the policies, as well as tactics to maximize revenue and fairly compensate physicians.

PHYSICIAN COMPENSATION CHECKLIST

General Readiness

- ☐ Establish profit centers for non-FFS accommodations such as call centers.
- ☐ Assess costs of accommodations for non-FFS arrangements such as clinical standards, documentation tools, CEHRT setup, and patient education.
- ☐ Develop general physician compensation guidelines for each non-FFS type, addressing the calculation of funds to be distributed and the mechanism based on the timing of services and payments.
- ☐ Create policy for compensating physicians for strategic and tactical support for non-FFS based services.

Non-FFS Plan Setup

- ☐ If possible, negotiate terms and conditions within the current capabilities of the practice/HCO.
- ☐ Assess non-FFS requirements and determine any changes to staffing, operations, and technology costs.
- ☐ Determine the costs that should be allocated to the plan before distribution of revenue to providers.
- ☐ Set up quality and operational requirements needed to support the non-FFS plan.

Operational Non-FFS Requirements

- ☐ Ensure that costs are being properly collected to support physician compensation calculation.
- ☐ Monitor provider activities to meet performance and quality standards for the non-FFS plan.

Manage Results

- ☐ Evaluate financial results for each non-FFS arrangement, including cost allocations and patient service requirements.

CHAPTER 3

Tools of the Trade: Practice Management Systems

Hundreds of FFS-focused practice management and medical billing system vendors have been working on the challenges and problems of FFS-based healthcare for over 40 years. However, these FFS tools do not directly address the plethora of non-FFS arrangements or even the nuances between the different non-FFS arrangements that you may be dealing with. As important, many non-FFS arrangements require more intense coordination of CEHRT and PMS information than the typical FFS-based charge interface from the CEHRT to the PMS. For example, your non-FFS contract may require certain clinical activities within a set time for each patient assigned to the practice/HCO.

PMS products are focused on the FFS model. The master files, patient information, and features are designed to deal with the basic FFS issue for each individual claim and charge:

Standard Fee	$100
Less Reduction to Payer Usual and Customary	– $10
Less Contractual Write-Off	– $20
Equals Payer Approved Amount	$ 70
Less Payer Payment	– $56
Equals Patient Co-Payment	$14

Non-FFS relationships frequently include performance requirements and payment mechanisms that are loosely connected or not connected at all to a specific charge. A periodic non-FFS payment may be based on how the practice/HCO performs various quality and patient service requirements. Practices/HCOs must be careful to analyze how such services should be tracked as well as how the payments should be posted to maintain the integrity of clinical and financial records. Otherwise, the practice/HCO could be surprised to find that its efforts were not effective and its performance payments were not earned.

The challenge for the non-FFS environment is how to co-opt PMS features to address non-FFS business and management issues. The non-FFS relationship may require more plan-specific handling of patients and new tools. For example, the non-FFS arrangement may require use of a treatment and patient service strategy. In other non-FFS situations, your practice may need to develop new ways to encourage patients to achieve your performance goals and increase your own profits. For example, you may invest money in non-billable activities to monitor patients and earn a shared savings payment that exceeds your additional costs.

The following strategies should be considered in how you use your PMS in the non-FFS environment:

Charge Codes

Charge codes (sometimes called service codes) contain the CPT® codes used by the HCO/practice as well as a standard fee for each charge. In some cases, the RVUs and even a cost can be assigned to a charge. Many FFS analytical reports and tools are based on the differences between the standard charge and the revenue received. For example, PMSs produce a report of realization (payments received divided by charges) by payer, as well as by charge code by payer.

Since charge codes are the key to so many PMS and CEHRT capabilities, charge codes are critical to managing non-FFS arrangements. Using practice/HCO-created charge codes outside of the CPT® codes utilizes features of the PMS and CEHRT to support important non-FFS activities:

Track contacts with patients. The non-CPT® codes would be set up for various activities such as initial consultation, follow-up discussions over the phone, and monitoring patient information for each type of position such as health coach or clinical call center nurse.

Track patient-level services. PMS and CEHRT tools can identify patients who have not recorded a specific non-CPT® service within the required parameters of the contract. For example, the practice/HCO could produce a list of patients who have not had a telemedicine consultation in the last four weeks.

Additionally, non-CPT® charge codes could be used to record a web-enabled spirometer supplied to a patient as well as a second non-CPT® charge code for patient follow-up on spirometer readings.

The absence of a charge code from a patient record may indicate that staff members need to follow up on a treatment or order.

Determine value services for analysis. The charge codes could be used to determine the value of services provided to patients under a non-FFS structure. The value of services could be deducted from revenue before allocating the net non-FFS revenue to physicians.

A standard cost for patient services could be assigned to non-FFS activities such as non-physician staff activities through a clinical call center. A different non-CPT® charge code could be used (with a different cost) for each type of clinical staff (i.e., medical assistant, nurse, PA). The charge codes could be the basis for a report that calculates costs and utilization.

Trigger clinical decision support (CDS). CDS interventions are a fail-safe patient care standard. For example, some CEHRTs could trigger an intervention for a patient on a non-FFS care management plan that had not had a counseling session in a week.

> *CAUTION:* The CDS feature can be used as a fail-safe, but patient-specific orders should be used to fine-tune patient service and care.

Payment and Adjustment Codes

PMSs use payment and adjustment codes to post receipts to charges as well as adjust charges for contractual write-offs, bad debts, and other credits. Some include information about whether the adjustment is a credit or a debit adjustment. Adjustment codes will be needed to accommodate incentive and performance payments that are not associated with a patient as well as deal with posting of unbilled charges to the patient account. For example, you may have an adjustment code to write off charges that are not billed to the non-FFS payer but represent real practice/HMO expenses.

The cumulative adjustment code value could serve as a benchmark to measure the profitability and realization of non-FFS incentive payment. For example, the practice/HCO may have received a $13,550 payment for care management, but incurred $8,500 in charges for staff to work with patients on care issues. The remaining non-FFS revenue could be allocated to physicians.

Some PMSs cannot accommodate payments that are not associated with a claim. Others will allow you to post a payment to an adjustment code. For example, a shared savings payment may be posted to an adjustment code (such as ADJSS1 for Adjustment for Shared Savings Insurance Company 1) that is also used to write off charges (such as patient adherence counseling) for a shared savings arrangement. This strategy would capitalize on the PMS productivity reports to track the shared savings net revenue.

If the PMS does not support the use of adjustment codes, the practice/HCO could generate a report of the shared savings activity by payer and export the information to a spreadsheet to complete the revenue analysis. Alternatively, the practice/HCO could use one adjustment code for the payment and a second code for the charge write-offs associated with non-FFS costs. Reports on the charges by charge code could be used to compare payments with the service costs.

> TIP: Regardless of the handling of unbilled charges, the practice/HCO needs to track the level of effort for non-FFS plan realization analysis.

Payers and Plans

PMS payer files may manage multiple plans under the payer. Payer information includes address, billing, and contact information, as well as selected plan terms such as referral authorization requirements and fee schedules.

The practice/HCO may have more than one distinct arrangement with a payer. If the PMS payer file does not accommodate plans, a separate payer record would be needed for each relationship. For example, you may need a payer record for FFS claims and another payer record for the non-FFS care management arrangement.

TIP: Many PMSs allow you to set up a group of payers to combine payers for reporting purposes. For example, you could set up a payer group for all Blue Cross Blue Shield non-FFS plans.

Non-FFS arrangements are profiled with important details, including treatment requirements and allowed services. Some PMSs allow for explanatory notes to make the key details available to administrative and clinical staff. Additionally, some PMSs allow for payer-specific allowed charge codes. For example, the payer charge codes could be limited to the covered services in the non-FFS contract and selected non-CPT® codes for patient service tracking. Thereby, non-FFS charge codes for remote patient monitoring system (RPM) devices could be excluded for non-FFS plans that do not include an RPMS in the care management fee.

TIP: If a note area is not available, you may create an online document or chart summarizing the key issues and requirements for each non-FFS arrangement.

Payer Fee

Payer fee tables include the payer-specific and, in some cases, plan-specific charges and expected payments as well as billing instructions. For example, some PMSs allow you to block a CPT® code from billing to a payer.

Payer fees tables should be carefully structured for the non-FFS arrangement to track services for patient care and cost purposes. For example, an unbillable charge, such as a call center consultation, could be assigned an expected fee of 0, but a charge of $15 to track activity and costs at the patient level.

Some PMSs immediately write off fees that will not be billed to the payer. The PMS will generate two transactions (the charge and the write-off) for each unbillable charge. Practices/HCOs should set up a specific write-off code (such as NONFFSREQ) that will isolate the non-FFS activities for each payer. Otherwise, it may be difficult to analyze the performance of non-FFS arrangements. For example, separate write-off codes should be used for contractual write-offs, non-FFS covered services, and performance penalty adjustments. Thereby, the practice/HCO can track the lost revenue due to not meeting performance standards as well as costs associated with unbilled patient services.

> *ALERT:* If the write-off codes cannot be isolated for each payer and plan, you may have to create a distinct code for each non-FFS arrangement such as CONTRWOBCBS, and CONTRWOMCARE.

Charges and Claims

CPT® code entry serves important purposes outside of billing. For example, charges may trigger CDS interventions, identify patients who require a time-critical procedure, and allow practices/HCOs to determine the number of patient-provided services. In many non-FFS situations, the entry of a CPT® code is not related to billing or payment. For example, a practice may submit a special CPT® code to be paid for an episode of care. However, recording unbillable codes for the services under the episode of care may be critical to track performance, patient care, and costs.

Many PMSs allow you to block claim submission for a specific charge code at the charge, payer, and/or plan level. The ability to block billing of any charge code used for tracking services provided under non-FFS arrangements is an important tool to support non-FFS analysis and patient service. In that way, non-FFS revenue can be evaluated in context with practice/HCO patient service efforts and costs.

In some cases, payers require reporting of the CPT® charges for non-FFS activities through the claim-submission process. Claims for services covered under the non-FFS arrangement may require a zero charge to report on services, depending on the payer. For example, a payer may want to track immunizations for patients under a capitated plan.

Charges that are billed to non-FFS payers can be submitted for payment through the standard claim process.

Payment Posting

PMSs are designed primarily to post payments to outstanding claims on a line-item basis. Many non-FFS payments are not connected to a claim and pose several challenges, including:

- Periodic payments may be paid for the previous or a future period. If a payment is for the following month, the analysis of performance and services may not be accurate until several weeks after the payment is received.

- The practice/HCO may not know the payment amount until the payment is received. For example, a performance payment based on ranking with other HCOs in the Accountable Care Organization (ACO) would yield a payment that was not determined or submitted by the practice/HCO.
- Payments may apply to a large group of patients being served with varying levels of services and needs covered under the non-FFS contract. For example, some patients may have frequent contact with the practice since the remote patient monitoring systems trigger alerts for weight gain by some patients while other patients are more successful controlling their weight.

Payments may be paid for activities that may or may not be associated with specific patient procedures. For example, a shared savings payment may not be connected to any specific patient CPT® charges although the practice may have performed services to achieve the savings. Also, practices/HCOs dedicated to raising patient awareness and adherence may result in cost savings from patients following evidence-based medical strategies.

Since many non-FFS payments are based on a variety of factors, the practice/HCO will need to verify any non-claim-based payments received. For example,

- Performance payments should be verified with statistics maintained by the practice/HCO. For each non-FFS arrangement, the practice/HCO should develop strategies and tactics to ensure that patients are served and services are provided within the non-FFS requirements. The tracking strategy should yield information and statistics that can be used to verify the non-FFS plan information as well as help the practice meet performance thresholds. For example, the practice/HCO may produce a monthly report of patients who have not had an annual physical and contact the patient through a secure message to the patient portal.

> *TIP:* If a patient refuses to have a physical, the practice/HCO should document the refusal and use the information to work with the non-FFS sponsor to avoid being penalized in the calculation of incentives.

- Payments based on number of patients served should be verified with the information in the PMS and CEHRT.

> *TIP*: Verifying patient counts may require generating reports at the end of the relevant period, since counting covered patients afterwards may be difficult or impossible due to changes in coverage.

> *TIP*: To reconcile payments based on number of patients, the practice should review patients who changed coverage around the cut-off dates of the payment to ensure the patient counts are correct.

- Prospective payments based on a list of patients provided to the practice/HCO may require adding new patients to the PMS/CEHRT for new assignments as well as removing patients who are no longer covered. As important, the practice/HCO may be required to make initial contact or perform an initial consultation with a patient. For example, the practice/HCO may need to complete an initial assessment within two weeks of patient assignment.

> *TIP*: Consider using the patient portal for initial information from a newly assigned non-FFS patient. For example, the practice/HCO could develop a patient portal form for new patients based on the specific focus of the non-FFS arrangement.

Few PMS systems deal directly with the non-FFS payments outside of the typical claim structure. For reasons discussed throughout this book, the practice/HCO needs to track the CPT® and non-CPT® services provided to non-FFS patients. The general strategy is to create non-FFS charge codes and post non-FFS charge codes as the patient is served without triggering a claim. Depending on the capabilities of your PMS and how the practice/HCO uses the PMS, the non-FFS charges may be immediately written off, posted as a zero charge, or posted with a fee for tracking purposes.

> *TIP*: If the non-FFS charge is posted with a fee, the fee should be written off to the non-FFS tracking code. Otherwise, the practice/HCO may be better off posting the charge with a zero amount and generating a report of non-FFS charge codes priced at the cost or some other relevant value.

If possible, the practice/HCO should set up their non-FFS strategy to natively track plan clinical and financial performance within the PMS.

That way, the plan can be reviewed throughout the month with standard PMS reports in real time. Otherwise, the practice/HCO may have periodic snapshots that may delay response to a problem that could limit revenue opportunities. Depending on the PMS and its use, the practice/HCO has several non-FFS payment posting options:

Post payments to a dummy patient record. In some cases, the non-FFS service payment is posted to a separate dummy patient set up for each non-FFS arrangement. The payment would be posted using the relevant adjustment code used to write off unbilled services required by the non-FFS arrangement. Therefore, the PMS reports can report on the net revenue of the plan offset by the value of the services provided.

Post payments to the services covered by the non-FFS plan. Some PMS vendors recommend posting non-FFS charges to the patient and then posting the non-FFS payment to the outstanding charges by patient. This method may distort the patient account, since outstanding charges will clutter up the patient account and may complicate figuring out the patient balance for most non-FFS arrangements. For example, the current patient balance may be difficult to determine among the outstanding charges that are covered by a case payment. As important, the charges could distort summary accounts receivable reports. The charges would inflate accounts receivable until "paid off" with the posting of the non-FFS payments.

This method does require some research, since the payment will not necessarily match the value of the services. If the payment is less than the value of the services, post the payment as a percentage of the total charges (i.e., $1,000 in charges with a $900 payment would be posted at 90% of the fees and the remaining amount written off to the adjustment code for the plan). If the payment exceeds the charges, then the charges would be fully paid and the remaining amount would be posted to the adjustment code used to write off charges for the specific non-FFS plan. A net report on the adjustment code would report on the comparison between the payments and the posted charges.

> *CAUTION:* This tactic can be time-consuming, since there may be many affected charges.

Post payments outside of the PMS. Many PMS products recommend posting payments not related to a claim outside of the PMS and into the accounting system. The following issues should be noted:

- If the practice/HCO does post non-FFS payments outside of the PMS, any realization report involving the non-FFS plans will be distorted. Therefore, the practice/HCO should isolate FFS plans from non-FFS reporting.
- If the practice does not post the non-FFS payments in the PMS, then multiple relationships with a payer could be distorted in PMS reporting. For example, a reduced FFS arrangement with non-FFS incentives would not be reflected in the PMS reports.

> *TIP:* If the practice/HCO must post the payment outside the PMS, the charge information could be exported to a spreadsheet program to document the plan payment and realization analysis.

> *CAUTION:* The best non-FFS posting strategy for your practice will depend on your PMS and how you use it.

> *ALERT:* Your payment-posting strategy and your ability to monitor performance will depend on the alignment of your payment-posting strategy with the non-CPT® charge codes discussed above.

Regardless of the payment-posting strategy used, the practice/HCO will need a mechanism to monitor the payment and analyze the performance considering the practice efforts, and the costs of meeting the non-FFS requirements.

Performance Reporting

Non-FFS analysis will vary by the type of arrangement. The basic strategy noted above would use the charge codes (including non-CPT®) to recognize the non-billable services provided to a patient. From the patient-level charges, the practice can analyze clinical and financial results. For example, a report of patient charges by non-FFS plan could be used to determine the value of the charges compared to the received payment.

> *CAUTION:* Although you may be able to drill down into more granular views of results, practices/HCOs must be careful

about context. For example, a visit, episode of care, and capitation analysis at the lowest level, such as a patient visit, may not be meaningful, since the arrangement may be set up to average out. For example, one expensive episode of care outlier may be offset by a surplus from many other episodes.

Reporting features can vary dramatically by PMS. However, the number of services can be reported from the PMS and exported to a spreadsheet or analytics tool for reporting and analysis. For example, a report summarizing the number of services by code could be generated for patients, payers and plans, providers, and time periods for export to an analytics tool if the PMS reporting tools are not sufficient. Once the analytics tool has been selected and interfaced for downloading information, the process can be repeated monthly.

Practices/HCOs should work to maintain information that can be used to justify their added value to the non-FFS payer. For example,

- Hospitalization rates and average cost of care compared to local averages or the experience of the HCO/practice with FFS populations would help verify the value of the non-FFS strategy.
- Clinical call centers may help avert unnecessary urgent care and emergency room visits based on classification of the problem and level of service provided to the patient.
- To generate the appropriate information, the practice should analyze the metrics that should be tracked for each non-FFS arrangement and design the patient service process to collect the relevant information. For example, a non-CPT® charge representing a new non-FFS patient intake interview over the phone could be used to track the value of services provided as well as prove that practice/HCO has been onboarding patients within the non-FFS performance standard.

> *TIP:* Practices/HCOs should go beyond the minimum tracking requirements to include metrics and statistics that highlight performance. For example, time to respond to a patient secure message may not be in the non-FFS contract, but such a statistic would highlight patient service and the practice's/HCO's investment in staff and processes around the patient portal.

Patient service obligations and how the practice will pay for them is an emergent issue and requirement. Using the outstanding patient order information from the CEHRT, the practice/HCO can price the obligations by patient, non-FFS plan, and payer. The use of outstanding services will vary by type of situation. For example, in episode of care situations, the outstanding obligations will provide you with the level of service and costs that need to be covered by the EOC fees. The practice may want to reserve money to pay for the outstanding fees from advance payments or use the information to calculate the unencumbered funds for distribution to providers.

Appointment Scheduling

Appointment scheduling modules of PMSs are designed mostly for office visits. The appointment is assigned to a resource to track and manage office flow. The practice/HCO may want to use appointment scheduling to ensure that patient treatment is proceeding as recommended by the doctor. For example, some PMSs can associate an appointment with an order such as a lab test due to the patient condition or a service requirement driven by the non-FFS agreement. Ideally, the PMS appointment should be linked to the CEHRT-based patient order and clinicians should be able to determine the appointment status of a patient order from the CEHRT.

CHAPTER 4

Tools of the Trade: Electronic Health Records

Many CEHRTs are focused on the FFS environment. Their main purpose is to produce an encounter note that supports the billing of the Evaluation and Management Level Service on the claim. For non-FFS, you need to take full advantage of the CEHRT tools to track patient care and performance.

> *CAUTION:* You may need to challenge your CEHRT vendor to enhance its products to address your non-FFS needs. Otherwise, you could end up with a variety of workarounds and tracking systems outside of the CEHRT that would undermine your operation and stymie your non-FFS efforts. For example, some practices post patient service items to a standard Outlook calendar.

Under non-FFS arrangements, resources are needed to guide and manage the patient outside of the clinical visit. Some of these activities will help patients avoid office visits, home health visits, and even hospital stays. As important, the specific details of each non-FFS plan may affect the treatment and patient service options. For example, some care management plans may pay for group meetings and online logs through your website.

Each non-FFS relationship must be analyzed to determine the responsibilities of the practice and patient service strategy. The practice/HCO will proceed to design an effective way to meet the non-FFS requirements as well as track performance and results. The practice/HCO will need non-FFS supporting CEHRT features to address important issues, including:

Clinical Content. Clinical content consists of the CEHRT forms, checklists, and other items specific to the area of medicine. For example, a patient portal intake form, initial patient intake for a diabetes patient, and the template for a follow-up visit are all examples of clinical content. A practice/HCO looks for relevant clinical content when purchasing a CEHRT.

The practice/HCO may need additional templates to document services outside of office visits. For example, the practice/HCO may need templates for the initial intake targeting non-FFS requirements, focused office visits, and clinical call center-based services. Indeed, the full cycle of patient care must be accommodated to ensure that all patient services are presented within context. For example, the CEHRT will need effective tools to manage dialogues with patients through clinical call centers as well as the ability to view call center services as part of the cycle of care that includes procedure documentation, encounter notes and periodic patient surveys.

Patient Education. Patient education should be redesigned to address the objectives and patient care issues associated with the non-FFS plan. General disease and treatment information should be replaced with more specific information relevant to the target population as well as explain treatment strategies and protocols that may be specific to the non-FFS plan. For example, the practice/HCO may:

- Include lifestyle advisories within the treatment strategy for a non-FFS arrangement;
- Offer non-FFS plan-specific treatment and care strategies that need supporting patient education;
- Present online videos to demonstrate physical therapy exercises for specific issues and problems; and/or
- Develop targeted patient education information about specific disease stages that apply to the patient rather than general information and broader disease states that may confuse the patient.

The practice should verify that the patient education is strategically aligned with the patient's treatment strategy as well as the clinical standards that have been established by the practice/HCO under the non-FFS plan.

Since electronic patient education is an Advancing Care Information measure, the practice/HCO may also consider investing in a wider range of patient education tools. For example, videos may be developed to demonstrate how to use a piece of equipment or explain a procedure.

Treatment Plans. Non-FFS arrangements generally increase the responsibility of the practice/HCO for patient adherence. Payments may be based on quality issues as well as performance measures that ensure patients receive treatment and services to improve or maintain patient health. Similarly, treatment plans and patient management are an important tool to generate savings for a shared savings plan.

Treatment plans typically are composed of one or more CEHRT orders. Treatment plans and orders are extensively discussed in Chapter 5—Tools of the Trade: Orders.

The following sections review the important features needed to succeed in the non-FFS environment for the CEHRT and significant modules related to the CEHRT.

Electronic Health Records

Visit Notes

The visit note is designed to produce a valid evaluation and management (E&M) to support your FFS bills. Under non-FFS, significant interactions with patients outside of office visits will need to be documented. Under FFS, just about all activities are geared to culminate in an office visit or a procedure. Therefore, ancillary activities and patient contacts are not necessarily considered or presented as part of the clinical care strategy. For example, many CEHRT products do not consider messaging part of the patient medical record. Similarly, patient recall tools in the PMS are not even available through most CEHRTs, and some patient portals do not post patient messages to the CEHRT.

In the non-FFS environment, a wide array of activities outside of the office visit are significant patient service events that need to be tracked and presented in context to monitor patient issues and status. For example, a bi-weekly check on patient status and daily report on glucose levels need to be accessible and presented in the patient record. In many systems, key non-FFS activities are not easily accommodated outside of creating an encounter note. For example, some CEHRTs present daily blood pressure readings in an encounter note that cannot be viewed or graphed for trend analysis. In many cases, diagnostic reports are passed to CEHRTs as images that are not searchable or discretely noted in the patient record.

> *TIP:* If your CEHRT does not include patient messages as part of the patient record, consider other documentation options such as a clinical note and patient orders. If your CEHRT does include patient messages as part of the patient record, consider using a standard set of message descriptions (i.e., PA consult over phone, alert message for abnormal glucose) to clearly display the nature and context of non-FFS activities. For example, scale-reading follow-up, patient-initiated telemedicine consultation, and office-initiated telemedicine consultation may be standard message topics. Some CEHRTs accommodate a message template. For example, the practice may set up message templates to accommodate a health coach or counseling telemedicine session with a patient.

The visit note feature is an important tool to record non-FFS encounters, but the practice/HCO needs to standardize the use of notes for each type of patient service. For example,

- Establish different note formats for each type of non-office visit, such as clinical call center encounters, telemedicine visits, and remote patient monitoring information. If appropriate, the practice/HCO may set up different note formats to address the focus of different plans. For example, a patient may be encouraged to participate in exercise classes offered by the plan sponsor.
- Differentiate the non-office visits from office encounters. Non-office patient services may have specific objectives and protocols that are important to monitor and serve patients. For example, some CEHRTs accept a short description or encounter type that could be used to differentiate various types of non-FFS patient services when viewing the list of contents. A report writer may report on the number of office encounters with a specific description, or the last time an office note description occurred in a patient record.

TIP: If the CEHRT does not support differentiation of office notes, you may be able to use the non-FFS service code to quickly identify the type of note and patient service. For example, posting a non-CPT® charge code of "health coach follow-up" will differentiate the note, and help the practice/HCO track productivity and costs.

Presentation of Information

The CEHRT patient summary screen presents key information from the complete record. Patient summary screens may display medications, lists of encounters, diagnoses, patient orders, and other items. CEHRT presentation options include filters to select displayed information and sort order option by date or reverse date order. For example, you can filter out expired prescriptions or completed orders.

For non-FFS, the outstanding patient issues and treatment plan with status is important. From shared savings to quality-based incentives, the staff and physicians are constantly seeking ways to monitor and respond to evolving patient issues and ensure that patients follow the treatment recommendations. Indeed, any contact with a patient is an opportunity to check in on patient status and remind patients about treatment issues.

The patient summary screen should help physicians and staff isolate documentation on different types of services and quickly access useful views of information. For example, looking at current messages is important, but viewing all services in chronological order may help uncover important trends. For example, the doctor may want to see the sequence of patient service events to study the office visit encounters within the context of health coach sessions or focus on the health coach sessions.

Clinical Decision Support Interventions

CDS interventions were a Meaningful Use requirement; they are not included in the Advancing Care Information requirements for MIPS. CEHRT products use a variety of strategies to address CDS rules or interventions. At a minimum, the CDS options are driven by drugs, drug allergy, demographics (such as age and gender), vital signs, and lab tests/results. Some CEHRT products also allow CDS interventions to be triggered with procedures and even specific medical note findings. For example, some CEHRTs allow you to trigger the intervention based on a high pain level. The clinical decision intervention feature can be repurposed for non-FFS.

CDS can be used to create intervention rules that can act as a backstop to catch patients who may not have an appropriate order (see Chapter 5). For example, a CDS intervention may be set up for annual exams for hip replacements. Some CEHRTs allow a useful degree of granularity. For example, you may be able to trigger a clinical to-do for patients covered by the non-FFS payer who have not called the clinical call center within a month.

> *ALERT:* Even though CDS is useful, physicians should enter the relevant orders for the patient's situation and other clinical factors. For example, a patient with other issues at risk may be brought in every six months rather than the CDS-mandated 12 months. However, CDS driven by the non-FFS arrangements (some CEHRTs can include payer plans in the CDS rule) will ensure that all relevant patients are properly managed and served. For example, for a specific non-FFS plan, the practice/HCO may set up CDS rules based on the non-FFS care standards.

> *CAUTION:* Some CEHRTs present CDS interventions separately from orders entered for the patient or in a mechanism outside of the patient service process. For example, some CEHRTs display CDS intervention analysis in a supplemental popup that indicates the patient status for all CDS rules. The popup must be selected and the list analyzed for relevant patient service issues. Users would have to specifically access the CDS feature to view the patient advisory.

Messages

CEHRT messages are used to track patient issues and clinical work. Messages may be used to flag review of an incoming lab report, document a patient call, or notify a staff member to call a patient. Some CEHRTs do not consider messages as part of the patient record and other CEHRTs always consider messages as part of the patient record. Some CEHRTs allow the user to select whether a selected message should be included in the patient record.

ALERT: CEHRTs that do not have an office flow tool use messages to notify staff about patient location and next steps. However, office routing messages clutter up the patient's clinical record and complicate tracking trends and intervening incidents between office visits.

Although the message capabilities vary between CEHRT products, the following message feature attributes may help document non-FFS efforts:

- Messages description or type. Message description or a type code (i.e., health counselor phone call, surgery education session) can be used to classify the message for tracking patient service trends and issues. For example, you may contact a patient who submits many portal questions to determine if the patient's health situation warrants a different patient service strategy.
- Message status. Many CEHRTs allow messages to be assigned a status such as open, closed, cancelled, and pending. Message status can be used to monitor messages and ensure messages are addressed on a timely basis. For example, the daily monitoring may verify that all refill request message types are responded to within a clinical session.
- Message templates. Message templates structure the information entered in a message. For example, different templates can be designed for a post-procedure secure message to a patient or a periodic telemedicine session.
- Attachments. Some CEHRTs allow messages to be directly attached to a relevant result, scanned document, or even a part of the patient medical record. For example, messages from a third-party patient portal required by an ACO can be loaded as a message attachment to become part of the clinical documentation.

> *ALERT:* Many CEHRTs do not support message attachments and the connection to the supporting message is obscured. For example, the message may reference the test result, but the user would have to find the image in the patient record separately. If the message is attached to the result, the user can click on the link to view the result.

Scanned Documents

Although more and more information is available electronically, images of reports and other clinical data will be in use for the foreseeable future. For example, radiology images, faxed reports, and patient records from other providers will continue to be scanned or loaded as an image into the CEHRT.

Some CEHRTs accommodate comments, notes, classification codes, and other information that may help describe and/or summarize the image. Ideally, the practice/HCO should be able to highlight important information on the image and attach one or more comments to highlight or explain information on the image.

Scanned documents may also be used to store any relevant patient notifications faxed to the practice/HCO from the non-FFS plan administrator or collaborating provider. The practice/HCO may need to abstract the scanned document into the patient record to ensure that the patient is properly treated. For example, a status report from the primary care provider may trigger a follow-up contact with a patient by a specialist who has released the patient back to the primary care practice.

Flow Sheets

Flow sheets present multiple findings and readings over time. In most CEHRTs, lab results can be viewed in a flow sheet format. Some CEHRTs also accommodate almost any information in a flow sheet. For example, patient responses to surveys, vital information, and readings from remote glucose meters may be saved in flow sheet format. A user can view the entries to look for trends and may be able to view relevant information on a graph.

> *TIP:* Many non-FFS strategies generate more patient contacts and information that may be managed most effectively through a flow sheet. For example, periodic patient portal care surveys and glucose meter readings may be analyzed more effectively in a flow sheet. Practices/HCOs should include a review of flow sheet candidates when planning their non-FFS patient service strategies. For example, use of RPM systems may require flow sheet tools to manage and analyze daily patient reporting.

Training

Although not a purely technical issue, training of doctors, providers, and staff in the use of practice/HCO systems, policies, and procedures will be needed to ensure that the organization uses the CEHRT as intended. As important, physicians and staff may need training on the specific requirements of non-FFS plans and how the practice/HCO addresses patient service, performance, and quality tracking.

> *TIP:* Consider using recorded web meetings to make training available to all staff at any time. For example, the practice may have a session on orders as well as how patient-driven delays should be reported to the non-FFS plan administrator.

Audit Trails

CEHRT requires an audit trail of any patient information change, access, and other activities. Depending on the CEHRT, the audit trail may be easily accessed from the relevant patient screen or through an audit trail access tool. For example, some CEHRTs allow you to see the specific changes to a prescription with the date, time, user, and change. Audit trails are useful to view the exact sequence of events for analyzing the patient situation or reviewing service-response efforts. For example, an audit trail could be used to measure the response time to a patient question submitted as a secure message over the patient portal.

Under an ACI measure, patient information is available electronically to patients. Most CEHRT products use a patient portal to provide electronic access. Practices/HCOs need to carefully consider how the information will be presented to the patient and interpreted by the patient. For example, illegible notations or test results without any directions or comments may confuse patients. In addition, presentation of extensive information without clear directions about the treatment plan and patient instructions may be useless to a patient.

> *TIP:* Include the presentation of information on the portal as part of the practice/HCO training to sensitize physicians and staff on the challenges that patients may face when accessing their information. Additionally, physicians and staff should be aware of how the entered information is presented to the patient. For example, physicians may improve the clarity of their messages to facilitate patient access to practice/HCO information.

Patient Service Tools

Patient service is a key challenge in the non-FFS environment. Success with non-FFS strategies requires more attention to providing advice and guiding patient issues outside of an office visit. Your non-FFS agreement or strategy may depend on effectively and frequently monitoring and working with patients. Indeed, the non-FFS strategies that you develop may be the key to better clinical and financial results.

The increasing importance of patient outreach requires that patient contact become an important part of the patient medical record. For example, some CEHRT systems use third-party patient portals that do not include patient portal exchanges as part of the patient's clinical record. As important, many CEHRT systems do not include general patient communications as part of the patient record, which can complicate monitoring patient wellness and care trends. Indeed, some practices/HCOs still record messages on papers that are scanned into the patient chart.

To capitalize on CEHRTs for patient service, you need management tools to facilitate identifying patient service issues and handling issues efficiently and effectively. For example,

- The patient summary screen should clearly highlight overdue-treatment orders and outstanding patient issues.
- The CEHRT should present a worklist of patients scheduled for follow-up services and calls. The HCO/practice should be able to view the list based on filters such as the type of service, due date, and provider. The worklist should include tools to record an interaction with a patient, send a secure message through the patient portal, document a discussion with a patient, and/or set up a follow-up tickler date.
- A patient service screen should display the status of expected remote patient monitoring reports from patients. Patient information that generated a remote patient alert should be accessible through a worklist tool.
- Practice/HCO managers should be able to quickly identify patient service issues older than a select period of time to monitor activities and address problems within the clinical session as well as during the day, week, and month.

Remote Patient Monitoring Tools

Remote patient monitoring (RPM) tools provide a stream of information about a patient's situation from a variety of dedicated devices and smartphone apps. Depending on the patient's condition, patient input may be objective readings or subjective information. For example, a web-enabled spirometer could be used by a patient on a periodic basis to track an asthma patient or the effectiveness of a change in medications. Similarly, patients could use a smartphone app to report on pain levels or attacks related to their condition.

A patient may use an RPM tool at any time of the day or night. As a practical matter, the incoming information should be monitored through a screening tool. RPM information is uploaded from the patient's device or smartphone into a cloud-based monitoring system. The cloud-based monitor measures the incoming information against rules that may be based on the specific patient, patient condition, or even trends.

If the incoming information triggers a rule, the clinical call center or other responsible party will be notified about the incident. For example, a patient-specific rule may trigger a warning to the physician if the patient pain level is not relieved in a 12-hour period. A physician may set a patient-level rule to issue an alert for a high glucose reading. General alert levels could be set for any glucose reading.

To further illustrate:
- A spirometer in the patient's home may be used to test the patient in the morning and at night.
- A scale would record a patient's weight daily.
- A glucose meter may report to a cloud-based monitoring system for each use.
- A smartphone app could collect answers to a health assessment question-naire on a periodic basis.
- A patient may receive a query on health status for failing to use a device or report his or her pain level within a 12-hour period (the reporting frequency would be another patient-specific rule).
- A patient could use a smartphone app to report on a GI attack related to IBD.
- A home-based blood pressure device may be used by patients at certain times during the day.
- Activity information may be uploaded to report on prescribed patient activity for each day.

RPM tools can track reporting frequency and patient contact. For example, the monitoring system could send a message to the patient's smartphone that the patient has not reported within 24 hours with a request to weigh themselves. If the patient does not respond, the monitoring system could send a message to the clinical call center to contact the patient directly.

RPM provides a history of the patient's situation and permits analysis of trends over time, including problematic increases in frequency or severity of the problem. Consequently, patient health reporting will be more timely and accurate rather than relying on anecdotal information from patients.

Depending on the non-FFS plan, a patient may be eligible or required to be enrolled in an RPMS strategy. For example, a care management program may include payments for using an RPMS for all patients covered by the program. In other instances, your practice/HCO may decide that RPMS tools could be used to achieve a lower cost for services based on an episode of care fee or as a strategy to earn a shared savings incentive.

Setting up RPMS requires the practice/HCO choose the needed devices or smartphone applications as well as the cloud-based tools to analyze and store incoming information. Depending on the payer arrangement, the payer may pay for the service directly or include the RPMS in your practice/HCO scope of work.

Provisioning RPMS services may involve ordering equipment to be delivered to the patient and/or installation of an app on their smartphone. The patient is set up in the RPMS cloud system and the service establishes communication with the patient's devices and/or smartphone. The patient-specific reporting parameters and triggers must be set up in the RPMS monitoring system. For example, the doctor may set up reporting frequency as well as alert levels for the patient.

Many CEHRTs and PMSs are not designed or equipped to directly support RPMS. The continual monitoring of incoming information and the trigger rules for patients and groups of patients are not handled by most CEHRT products. If a supplemental RPMS tool is used, the practice/HCO still needs to ensure that the complete patient-designated record is maintained and that all relevant patient information is available to support patient care. For example, the RPMS may send a periodic report to the CEHRT.

Remote Telemedicine Services

Patients may be served remotely through a HIPAA-compliant Skype or Gchat-like connection. Through telemedicine services, patients can be more actively managed and served. For example, a practice/HCO could contact a patient about the effect of a new medicine or recovery from a procedure. As important, patients who defer clinical services may be served through telemedicine strategies. This allows the practice/HCO to "stretch the clinic" and fulfill patient needs even if obstacles such as transportation problems or out-of-town trips prevent a clinical visit. Telemedicine tools allow you to monitor patient health and continuity of care regardless of logistical and timing challenges. For example, the clinical staff may be able to follow up on the status of a procedure site, skin issue, or degrees of motion, as well as other patient issues.

> *TIP:* Telemedicine presents a new patient service and revenue opportunity for patients who may spend extended periods of time out of the area. Such patients could still be monitored on a continuing basis and the practice/HCO would be able to more effectively manage and monitor patient care. For example, patients who move to Florida for the winter could continue to be served within appropriate clinical standards.

Unfortunately, many of the remote telemedicine services separate the communication with patients from service documentation. For example, the clinician separately documents the service in the CEHRT and captures a picture of a mole that the patient showed to the clinician during the telemedicine visit.

From a billing perspective, some telemedicine services may be billed under an FFS structure, included in a global episode of care payment or covered under a care management contract. Note that telemedicine services may be particularly effective in care management situations because short monitoring exchanges with at-risk patients may prove effective and ensure more accurate information on their disease status. For example, more frequent checking of a wound using telemedicine may be more effective and less expensive than an office visit weeks later or several home visits.

> *ALERT:* Using telemedicine services to serve patients with chronic diseases can also consume more staff resources

for patients who may be frustrated with their situation or isolated because of their health status. For example, a lonely patient may frequently initiate telemedicine services or extend their conversations with your staff beyond the time needed to address the clinical mission of your services. Consequently, telemedicine staff should be trained to deal with such situations while achieving the patient service objectives of the telemedicine visit.

TIP: Some payers pay practices for telemedicine services through a standard claim. In these situations, your practice/ HCO may be billing some telemedicine services through a FFS arrangement while other telemedicine services may be part of a non-FFS strategy.

Patient Portals

Patient portals offer another channel for patient engagement and monitoring. They provide a variety of information to patients about their current health status and history with the practice. Patient portals are used by most CEHRT vendors to provide electronic access to patient information under the Advancing Care Information component of the Medicare Merit-based Incentive Payment System. Patient portals can be accessed through computers, tablets, and even smartphones. Some patient portals have a smartphone-friendly interface.

For non-FFS arrangements, the key benefit of the patient portal is to highlight care recommendations, facilitate dialogue with patients, and provide relevant disease information. Some CEHRT vendors also use patient portals to gather RPM information.

In theory, patient portals provide access to patient information, but the presentation of patient information could be confusing and complicated. For example,

- Images available through the patient portal may not be accompanied by a clear explanation of the significance of the image and an explanation or note that the patient can understand.
- A patient may have to access numerous encounter notes to see the outstanding orders for the patient care.

- An encounter note dictated with speech-recognition software that includes a treatment plan will not be highlighted within the note or on the patient portal.

As important, if the practice/HCO is not using the CEHRT as designed, the patient portal will not necessarily present information in the right place. For example, if patient education is copied and pasted into the clinical note, the patient education information will not be separately displayed on the resources screen.

Patient electronic access to their medical records is a measure under the Advancing Care Information aspect of the MIPS. To support non-FFS objectives, practices/HCOs need to be able to highlight important information and comment on pertinent patient care issues. For any information posted to the patient portal, the practice/HCO needs to clinically vet the information (including incoming diagnostic results and scanned documents) to ensure that the information is properly presented and the patient properly informed. For example, many patient portals send an email to patients to note the posting of new information on the portal.

> *TIP:* The practice/HCO should check whether patients have reviewed important portal messages or information on a periodic basis.

> *ALERT:* The vetting of information prior to availability through the portal should ensure that the patient is contacted about important results before posting of information to the portal. Some CEHRT products automatically post patient information to the portal and expose the practice to patient service issues if the practice does not contact the patient first.

CHAPTER 5

Tools of the Trade: Orders

The "plan" part of a SOAP (Subjective, Objective, Analysis, and Plan) note is recorded in most CEHRTs as one or more orders. The plan may be as simple as a single order for an annual physical or consist of several orders to document a treatment plan. In many CEHRTs, orders are entered as a CPT® code with a due date. The CEHRT typically tracks the entry date.

Orders are a critical tool to manage and succeed with non-FFS arrangements and serve several important functions:

- **Manage Patient Care.** Orders track the specific actions that are needed to keep the patient well and/or improve their health. Orders may be driven by specific obligations for a non-FFS arrangement that compensates the practice for specific activities to speed care and save money. For example, periodic visits with patients may be required at different intervals for patients with various diseases and problems.
- **Document Disposition of Physician Due Diligence.** Since non-FFS payments may be based on patient service and care, the order-management function allows the practice/HCO to document clinical recommendations as well as the due diligence to ensure patient adherence. In the event of a patient compliance problem, such as patients who move out of the area for the summer or winter, the practice/HCO will have the data and information needed to explain patient adherence and treatment.
- **Track Performance Under non-FFS Arrangements.** Non-FFS programs have a variety of quality and performance requirements. The practice/HCO may report the results of the efforts or the payer may develop its own performance measures based on review of practice/

HCO information, patient surveys, and audits. Practices/HCOs should monitor their own performance in meeting response and care standards in the non-FFS agreement. The order information can be used to address lapses on a timely basis as well as measure the performance of the practice/HCO. For example, an ACO denied a performance incentive for vaccines due to the way the ACO calculated the measure. However, the practice/HCO produced its own data with supporting information that proved that the vaccine performance exceeded the ACO requirement.

- **Project Expenses for Patient Treatment Obligations.** For non-FFS arrangements, such as episode of care, orders represent an outstanding direct or indirect financial obligation. For example, the ability to manage orders may have a significant impact on a shared savings payment. In such cases, the practice/HCO may need to quantify the financial obligations for services that are not incurred at the same time as the relevant payment. For example, an episode of care fee may be received for a patient that will pay for services over several months. The outstanding orders allow the practice/HCO to track the outstanding costs to be covered in the future. Such information may be used to establish reserves to pay future bills or distribute physician compensation in sync with patient services.

To manage your non-FFS responsibilities, consider additional (non-CPT®) codes to track other responsibilities and programs. For example, the practice/HCO may use a non-CPT® code to line up patients for RPM or periodic check-ins. Similarly, you may set up a patient status check-in order for a health coach that may differ from a code from a nurse or PA. When entering a set of orders (possibly a treatment plan), the due dates will be used to properly set up the order sequence. For example, you may have several test orders followed by a two-week pause before therapy starts and a month delay before the procedure.

Under non-FFS arrangements, patients who are under continuing care should have an outstanding order for their next clinical activity. The next order may be for an annual checkup or a colonoscopy in 10 years. The next clinical steps may include a complex set of orders for treatment of a problem or a single continuing order to follow up with a monthly telemedicine visit. Analytical tools can be used to monitor patient orders as well as work with the plan sponsor on quality of care and supporting evidence-based medical strategies.

Patient orders represent the clinical recommendations of the physician to maintain and/or restore patient health. Once the doctor has entered and communicated a treatment plan consisting of one or more orders, the patient has been notified of the doctor's recommendation, but many practices/HCOs do not follow through on the disposition of the orders with patients under FFS models. For example, a patient with a kidney stone may be told to return for a follow-up appointment and test in a year, but many practices do not contact the patient to reinforce the treatment plan after the original visit.

Many non-FFS situations depend on and compensate the practice/HCO for guidance and encouragement of the patient to adhere to the treatment plan. Practice/HCO guidance may be required to earn or be included in non-FFS compensation. For example,

- An ACO contract may contain a performance measure for ensuring patients receive therapy. Patient adherence may be directly tracked with various quality and performance measures that affect payments.
- Using the order plan under the clinical best practices determined by the practice/HCO may lead to shared savings revenue or saving money from an episode of care fee. For example, pre-procedure therapy and/or counseling may have been proven to speed patient recovery and save money.

Unfortunately, many CEHRT order features will disappoint you in supporting non-FFS requirements. As important, failure to use the patient order feature may prevent the practice/HCO and patients from non-FFS program benefits. For example, if the doctor does not establish an order for periodic patient contact, then the CEHRT will not display the outstanding treatment order on the patient summary screen and the patient will not be listed on the overdue contact worklist screen.

Proper non-FFS order management requires a comprehensive and flexible order status. Unfortunately, many CEHRT systems track basic status information on an order such as ordered, completed, and cancelled. Many FFS issues cannot be properly managed with such a limited order status, but in the non-FFS arena, the handling and management of orders may have a direct impact on meeting contractual obligations and how you are paid. In fact, limited order management could prevent you from proving that the terms of the non-FFS program were met and may produce insufficient proof of due diligence by the practice/HCO in managing patient services.

The practice/HCO will need information to substantiate fulfillment of the non-FFS arrangement. As important, tools to analyze the realization and obligations of such non-FFS situations are essential. Order status documents the disposition of a patient order and the sequence of patient services and interactions to encourage patients. These efforts directly impact performance, quality, and income. Order-status issues include:

Open Orders. An open order is an order that has been newly entered for a patient. The open order should specify the service (such as a CPT® or non-CPT® code), desired start date, recommended completion data (for strategies that may take time such as therapy and RPM), and the responsible party. For example, you may refer the patient to another provider for a service that needs to be performed within a clinically driven period. In many CEHRT systems, the order stays open until it is closed or cancelled.

Scheduled Orders. In non-FFS situations, completion of the order within the care parameters may be a critical performance criteria. Therefore, the order needs to be associated with an appointment. Such scheduling may be with an internal or external resource. Ideally, the performing party should be associated with the order. Scheduling information may be needed to ensure that the practice/HCO receives or sends information on a timely basis under quality measures, such as the Closing the Referral Loop (PQRS 374) measure, and provides timely care under non-FFS standards. Additionally, the scheduling information allows the practice/HCO to know that the patient is on the road to adherence.

In-Process Orders. In-process orders are patient action items that are being actively worked on. For example, the practice/HCO may be waiting for a biopsy result or the surgical scheduling process may be in progress. The practice/HCO should maintain notes on the efforts to move the order forward.

Modified Orders. Orders may be modified for many reasons, including change in patient condition and clinically driven issues. For purposes of clarity, we are classifying a modified order as driven by the doctor and suspended order (see below) driven by the patient. Clinically driven issues and changes in patient conditions are continually used to fine-tune the treatment plan. Documenting the change reason and clinical response gathers information that could be analyzed for further improvements to patient service and cost control. For example, if physical therapy supplemented by telemedicine sessions with a physical therapy aide leads to faster recovery, then the analysis of the order changes could help quantify the effects and appropriate conditions.

Suspended Orders. Suspended or deferred orders pose a serious challenge to managing patients and documenting services. A suspended order is an order that has been changed due to a patient issue, even though the original order represents the clinical recommendation of the provider. The key issue is that a patient treatment plan recommended by the doctor may not be followed due to a patient issue. A patient may refuse or delay a treatment recommendation due to an economic issue, personal preference, or a scheduling issue.

The suspended order is technically overdue as far as the physician is concerned since the delay is not recommended by the physician and is driven by the patient. From a quality-monitoring perspective, the suspension is not based on the clinically based recommendation of the physician, but other factors that should not reflect on the quality of patient service or negatively impact any payer-specific performance issues. For example, a patient's decision to delay treatment until after a vacation is accommodating a patient desire, but should not negatively affect the practice's quality measure for serving the patient within a period.

> *ALERT:* Suspension information may be critical if a patient-driven change delayed treatment and exacerbated the patient's disease. For example, the documentation on the suspension may be used to address questions from a payer or other party regarding the reason for the delay and the practice's response. If the practice had cancelled the order or changed the due date, the records would have appeared to indicate that the physician had initiated the delay.

Cancelled Orders. Many CEHRTs allow orders to be cancelled; however, there are significant differences in the impact and importance of cancelled orders. As a practical matter, orders could be cancelled by the physician due to a change in patient health status such as the problem being resolved or the patient making progress more quickly than anticipated.

To properly track the order, the CEHRT should allow the doctor to enter a reason for the cancelled order such as eliminated due to patient progress. As noted above, cancelled orders should be properly evaluated by quality and patient service monitoring reports to avoid miscounting the number of patients who were not treated within guidelines and/or CDS interventions. For example, a CDS intervention could be triggered by the cancellation of an order when the patient problem list has not been updated to avoid triggering the CDS rule.

> *CAUTION:* Physicians should not cancel an order that is still part of the recommended treatment plan but has been refused by the patient as noted above under suspended orders.

Completed Orders. Completed orders were followed through to the successful completion and/or review. A completed order may be one step in a long process that included working with the patient through a diagnostic and/or treatment process.

Access to order history varies widely. Some CEHRTs bury order information in the audit trail while other CEHRTs display order statuses and change dates on the order screen. Under non-FFS programs, the history of the order and the relevant statuses may be needed to allow users to understand the patient service issues and initiate appropriate guidance and follow-up. The practice/HCO may need to review the progress and status of an order as well as evaluate meeting performance and quality standards.

> *TIP:* You may be able to work around an incomplete order feature by using comments with keywords that may be selected for review using a report writer. For example, you could structure an order note to include "Patient Change" or "Doctor Change." In other CEHRTs, an order note area may be used to document the history of the order.

Patient orders should be available at the patient and practice/HCO level. When you access the patient record, outstanding orders should be highlighted and overdue orders flagged. Considering the order-status discussion above, you should be particularly concerned about orders that are still recommended, but have not been performed due to a patient issue (referred to as suspended).

Order-management tools are needed to survey and follow up on outstanding orders for operational and patient service purposes. For example, the CEHRT should

- Provide a worklist of important overdue orders across all patients that meet a selection filter such as x-rays overdue or an important patient follow-up. The worklist feature should include tools to automatically contact the patient through the patient portal and/or allow the user to document a phone call or follow-up activity.
- Offer a worklist option to list patients that meet a CDS trigger to allow staff to review overdue-treatment rules.
- Provide a tool to review the list of active patients without an outstanding order to allow clinical staff to properly set the next clinical services for a patient. For example, the CEHRT should display a list of all diabetic patients who don't have an A1C scheduled.
- Accommodate a list of patients under a non-FFS payer and/or non-FFS plan that meet criteria based on clinical issues, diagnosis codes, and previous procedures. That way, the practice/HCO can verify that relevant patients are properly served within each specific non-FFS agreement. This capability may be important to identify patients who need additional orders or services due to a change in the treatment strategy driven by clinical issues or a change to the non-FFS arrangement. For example, a non-FFS plan may increase the care management fee to include remote weight management for obese patients.

Physicians and staff need to properly set up and enter the relevant orders for a patient that can be tracked. Providers who enter the treatment plan in a free-form text note or use ad hoc order descriptions that are not used by other physicians will prevent the staff and patient from being properly informed about the patient plan and situation. CEHRT features cannot analyze the free-form text note and analytical reports will not properly function. Indeed, your practice/HCO will not be able to monitor performance or prove the value of your services for non-FFS situations.

CHAPTER 6

Tools of the Trade: Clinical Call Centers

From proactive analysis of patient health status to facilitating patient treatment recommendations, contact with at-risk patients is more frequent and intense under the non-FFS models. Continuing attention to patient services will challenge most practices and healthcare organizations. The clinical call center is a critical tool to effectively and efficiently monitor and manage patients.

In many practices/HCOs, the patient service strategy is based on paper medical records. Typically, patient calls are taken by an answering machine, front desk staff, or triage staff. In many cases, the patient issues are recorded and passed to the doctor for an answer. In some cases, a triage line is staffed by nurses who offer basic information and advice to the patient and have the authority to manage the same-day appointments for the doctor.

In many cases, patient service strategies are managed within each location. For example, a practice with 10 offices typically has patient service staff in each location. The patient service process is a vestige of paper charts: patients cannot be served without being able to look at their chart. Indeed, some practices are creative about ensuring that patient service staff have the chart before talking to the patient. For example, some practices put the patient service staff in the middle of the medical records room so they can access the chart while speaking with the patient. In other situations, practices take messages or have the patient go to voicemail so the patient service staff can retrieve the patient chart before calling the patient back.

Often, practices/HCOs incur the cost of a clinical call center but do not benefit from the investment. For example, the 10-office practice mentioned above had 12 full-time staff (1 or 2 per office) dedicated to patient calls that added little to patient care, but controlled access to priority appointments. Practices in this situation may be able to create the clinical call center by redesigning the current process and relocating the current staff.

In other situations, the clinical call center will be an entirely new expense. For example, many practices/HCOs funnel all calls to the front desk staff to manage same-day appointments but offer no clinical advice. This strategy also keeps people in the office waiting to check in or out while the front desk staff addresses the phone traffic. In that situation, a call center would require new staff and space.

The non-FFS model changes everything about how practices serve patients through direct and indirect requirements that affect payments to the practice. Under some non-FFS arrangements, the practice has an incentive to control the cost of care using its own proprietary strategies and techniques. For example, an incentive payment may be tied to lower expenses which may be achieved with frequent non-physician contact with patients.

Evolving industry requirements also point to a call center strategy. For example, Advancing Care Information includes measures to gather information from patients outside of the clinical environment and use secure messages to maintain contact with patients. Regardless how patient issues get to the practice, the information must be triaged by appropriate clinical staff on a timely basis to assure that the patient is properly managed and served. For example, what good will remote patient information on their weight serve if no one is available to review the information outside of tolerances over the weekend?

If clinically appropriate, addressing patient issues without an office visit is allowed and encouraged under many non-FFS models. For example, a drug prescription can be refilled based on documenting a discussion with the patient over the phone, and a patient can be checked on through a Skype-like conversation with a clinical call center.

The clinical call center can address the explosion of real-time traffic from patients over the phone and over the Internet while freeing up the providers in the office to concentrate on the patients. As important, the clinical call center is instrumental in meeting patient care and services to earn and/or qualify for non-FFS revenue.

The clinical call center strategy addresses several important challenges:

- **Response to Patient Issues.** Many non-FFS arrangements include requirements to respond to patient issues on a timely basis. Such actions may be instrumental in providing effective patient care and avoiding unnecessary costs. For example, directing patients to a hospital if the doctor is not available may not be the most cost-effective or timely way to address a patient issue. These issues may evolve during business hours as well as outside of business hours. The current off-hours call strategy of connecting the patient with the doctor may prove inefficient and disruptive. For example, a constant stream of information from remote blood pressure devices may have to be analyzed 24/7. Interestingly, 24/7 access to clinical advice is a MIPS clinical improvement activity.

- **Patient Management.** Non-FFS arrangements may include incentives to proactively manage patient care and patient adherence to clinical recommendations. Such activities will require current information on patient treatment issues and strategies as well as tools to encourage patient adherence. Patient portals, outgoing patient calls, and monitoring overdue-treatment recommendations may be managed through the clinical call center. Additionally, any call to the clinical call center would be an opportunity to encourage adherence as well as raise awareness of treatment plans that need adjustment. For example, frequent patient calls and/or too many alerts from RPM systems may trigger an internal call center escalation to a mid-level provider in the call center.

- **Monitoring Patients.** A wide range of tools and processes are designed to more closely monitor patient care and status outside of an office visit. For example, payers may pay for telemedicine visits with patients by nurses and other professionals. Similarly, remote patient services may be part of home health visits, therapy programs, and patient-wellness strategies. For example, home health episodes of care that include call center checks with patients in place of home health visits are more cost-effective and convenient than home visits alone. Such strategies will increase in importance and require an organized strategy to address evolving patient issues without disrupting office clinical operations and physicians.

The clinical call center allows the patients and the practice/HCO to fully benefit from the instant access to patient information as well as more communication through the CEHRT, patient portals, and other tools to serve and monitor patients.

The key to effective clinical call centers is a structured and controlled process to establish, manage, and monitor patient issues. The following key issues should be addressed:

Call Center Tools

Many CEHRT products lack the tools to effectively manage a clinical call center. CEHRT limitations include the lack of management tools to track and assign issue flows from patient portals, incoming calls, incoming readings from remote devices, and even incoming referrals. Call centers also require routing and coordinating incoming calls to the available call center staff. Such requirements may be handled by your phone system.

In some cases, you may be able to create workarounds to support the call center or use software from a vendor allied with your CEHRT publisher. For example,

- CEHRT messages and/or clinical note tools may be used to structure, track, and document clinical call center activities.
- A third-party RPM system may be needed to monitor patient subjective and objective information submitted from patient homes or through smartphones.
- Third-party patient portal software may be used separately to manage and monitor incoming messages and even remote patient information. Patient portal software programs have varying degrees of interfacing with their CEHRT partners.

Operational and Clinical Protocols

The practice/HCO medical leadership should develop supporting clinical and operational protocols to frame and empower the call center services. Clinical standards should specify issues to be handled by the various call center staff as well as documentation templates customized for the situation and disease. Call center protocols should define the escalation strategy within the call center staff as well as physician monitoring of call center activities. For example, the problem type and/or patient health status determine whether the issue is managed by a nurse or PA, as well as triggers for immediately contacting the doctor on call.

The call center design will be built on the functional and clinical framework of the CEHRT. For example, the practice/HCO should verify that call center activities can be viewed and managed within the context of other clinical services and information.

The call center is a key strategic asset to support non-FFS requirements and enhance general patient contact and engagement under MIPS. In many cases, these capabilities will involve dramatic enhancements to current triage strategies or a new capability that requires new clinical guidelines and protocols.

Call Center Staff

The call center staffing requirements may differ dramatically from the current triage strategy. For example, many practices currently route all issues directly to the patient's doctor. Non-FFS strategies may require more clinically capable staff to advise and guide patients in an environment that will be receiving more information than current triage staff receive. Indeed, the call center may receive information at any time that could indicate a change in patient status and health risk without patient awareness. For example, the RPM information may indicate a problematic change in patient status that generates an alert message to the call center. Such a situation may trigger an immediate call to the patient to further assess the situation and initiate an appropriate strategy to mitigate a problem.

This centralized approach to triage and the development of staff capabilities as well as changes to practice/HCO cultures may take a fair amount of time and resources. For example, call center staffs can include PAs and LPNs as well as nurses to allow for escalation of patient issues within the call center. As important, the call center staff must develop a patient-oriented service culture that integrates with the rest of the practice/HCO operation.

Call Center Monitoring

Call center activities should be monitored to ensure quality and timely response. The monitoring function includes checking average response times, patient contact activities and patient service advisories, as well as providing physicians with proper notification of significant events and changes. Of course, all events should be documented in the patient's medical record.

Clinical call centers are an important tool to address the non-stop patient service and management needs of many non-FFS arrangements as well as accommodate the increased velocity and frequency of patient contact. However, call centers are not developed overnight and require an effective and clear clinical mandate driven by medical leadership as well as proper resources to fulfill its operational and patient service mandate.

CLINICAL CALL CENTER CHECKLIST

☐ Inventory sources and types of patient information received and sent by the call center such as secure messages, incoming documents, RPM information, and telemedicine sessions.

☐ Establish clinical standards for treatment and clinical advice available through the call center.

☐ Design staffing model and requirements.

☐ Implement CEHRT-based documentation tools for the clinical call center.

☐ Reassign and acquire staff to meet call center requirements.

☐ Train staff.

☐ Continuously monitor performance and issues.

CHAPTER 7

MIPS Adjustments

The Medicare Quality Payment Program under the final rules published in October 2016 offers two different mechanisms to earn money: Advanced Alternative Payment Models and the MIPS.

Advanced Alternative Payment Models

The Advanced Alternative Payment Model (AAPM) awards a 5% incentive payment to qualifying AAPM participants. To qualify, the AAPM must use a CEHRT, meet MIPS-like quality measures, and bear more than a nominal risk for financial losses. ACOs and shared savings models are possible structures for the incentive.

Other chapters in the book cover the non-FFS strategies that can support AAPMs and should be used to develop tactics to support the AAPM as well as earn the 5% Medicare incentive.

Merit-based Incentive Payment System

The Medicare MIPS combines the value-based modifier, Meaningful Use (now called Advancing Care Information), and the Physician Quality Reporting System (PQRS) into a single incentive system. The final components of MIPS are clinical improvement activities and cost.

Practices/HCOs or providers included in MIPS who do not fulfill the requirements will be forfeiting the opportunity to earn additional money. For the worst MIPS performers, Medicare will apply a negative payment adjustment starting at -4% in 2019 and increasing to -9% by 2022. On the other hand, providers who meet all MIPS requirements at a high level can earn a positive Medicare MIPS adjustment of up to 22% (12% maximum MIPS adjustment plus 10% exceptional performance) in 2019 and increasing to 37% in 2022, including the 10% exceptional performance bonus.

ALERT: Due to the changes in the 2017 requirements for 2019 adjustments, avoiding a negative adjustment is simple: report one quality measure and one clinical improvement activity. Therefore, the maximum positive adjustment of 12% may not be achieved if many providers meet the minimum requirements.

Key PMS Issues

MIPS adjustments pose serious financial and patient management challenges for your practice/HCO. Indeed, MIPS-adjusted payments could distort your performance and profitability. The key PMS issues follow.

Expected Payments. MIPS may have a substantial impact on Medicare payments. If your HCO/practice MIPS adjustment is based at the group level (a practice or HCO), then the MIPS-adjusted Medicare-expected payment is the same for all providers. If each individual provider is separately scored under MIPS, then a separate MIPS adjustment will be assigned to each provider, yielding a different expected payment for each provider and service combination.

Adjustment Handling. Under MIPS, a provider may have a negative or positive adjustment to the payment on a Medicare claim. Since the adjustments are tied to the FFS charges, MIPS adjustments could increase or decrease payments for Medicare services. For example, a $100 service claim could result in a payment between $96 and $122 in 2019 depending on the adjustment factor. The practice/HCO needs to decide whether the adjustment is treated as part of the expected payment or an additional bonus payment, as well as how the adjustment is treated for physician compensation.

CAUTION: Based on current Medicare claim processing, the claim amount would be written down to the Medicare reimbursement rate and the adjustment applied to the Medicare reimbursement rate. For example, if a claim for a service with a Medicare reimbursement of $100 were sent as a claim for $104 (expecting a +$4 (+4%) adjustment), the Medicare electronic explanation of benefits would include a $4 write-off of the claim amount to the Medicare reimbursement rate and add in a $4 adjustment.

ALERT: Monitor how your PMS vendor will deal with this change, since some PMS systems do not accept expected payments greater than the claim amount. Your PMS vendor may make changes to the calculation of the Medicare-expected amount that require more fee and payer setups as well as additional posting efforts.

MIPS Costs. MIPS efforts may increase costs for changes and improvements to meet clinical improvement, quality, and ACI requirements. The additional costs may not evenly benefit all practice/HCO providers. For example, some providers may not serve Medicare patients, or a practice may have providers that serve only pediatric patients. In some practices/HCOs, the MIPS-related expenses may be assigned to MIPS providers based on an allocation of expenses or perhaps an adjustment to their revenue-driven compensation. For example, you may adjust the percentage of physician compensation based on the additional resources and expenses of achieving a higher MIPS score.

MIPS Groups and Providers. Clinicians have two MIPS participation options: as an individual provider or as part of a group.

- For individual MIPS reporting, the MIPS score and adjustment will be provider-specific; thereby, a practice/HCO could have a different expected payment for each provider. For example, a $100 claim may generate a 2019 remittance of $96 for a provider who did not fulfill the minimum requirements, while another provider in that same practice who fulfilled all requirements could be paid $104.
- The group MIPS score represents the efforts of the entire group and the MIPS score and adjustment will be applied to the entire group. However, the HCO/practice may have some providers that fully support the MIPS requirements, as well as other providers that don't meet the performance requirements to attain a positive adjustment, but benefited from the group. For example, one provider in the group may not support MIPS but will receive a +$2 adjustment due to the group score. At the same time, the other providers may have earned a $4 adjustment (if individually evaluated), but will received the lower $2 adjustment due to the group score.

    TIP: The practice/HCO should set up an internal system to equitably allocate MIPS adjustments to providers based on each provider's MIPS performance. That way, high-scoring

MIPS providers are rewarded and low-scoring MIPS providers are incentivized to do better.

For example, the practice/HCO could allocate the MIPS incentive on a sliding scale based on the practice/HCO-calculated MIPS score for each provider. The actual allocation would be based on the provider's Medicare charges.

This strategy affects physician compensation, but not the billing or payment-posting strategy, since all providers in the group are assigned the same MIPS adjustment. For example, all providers in the practice/HCO would receive a +4% MIPS adjustment on the incoming payment, but provider allocations of the net adjustment for compensation purposes could range from -$4 to +$6.

Providers can be excluded from MIPS based on Medicare volume of less than $30,000 or less than 100 patients or participation in an AAPM.

Management Accounting

At the provider level, a negative MIPS adjustment is operationally comparable to a lower approved amount. However, the negative adjustment is not a contractual write-down, but a penalty for a poor MIPS score. Therefore, the MIPS adjustment value should be tracked with a different adjustment code than the contractual write-down. For example, A -4% adjustment works well with the standard PMS features as follows:

Practice Billed Amount	$108	
Less Billed Over Allowable Amount	$8	Medicare Allowed Write-off Code
Medicare Allowed Reimbursement	$100	
Less Co-Insurance	$20	
Less Minus 4% MIPS Adjustment	$ 4	MIPS Adjustment W/O Code
Net Medicare Reimbursement	$76	

A positive adjustment requires more planning and work. The disposition of a positive adjustment will depend on the provider compensation issues (Chapter 2) as well as any MIPS-related expenses allocations. For example,

Practice Billed Amount	$108	
Less Billed Over Allowable Amount	$8	Medicare Allowed Write-off
Medicare Allowed Reimbursement	$100	
Less Co-Insurance	$20	
Plus 4% MIPS Adjustment	+$4	MIPS Positive Adjustment Code
Plus 10% Exceptional Performance	+$10	MIPS Exceptional Performance
Net Medicare Reimbursement	$94	

The practice/HCO may decide to track and manage the MIPS adjustment components separately. For example, a practice/HCO may choose to credit the 10% MIPS exceptional performance adjustment to the best internal MIPS scores in the MIPS-scored group but allocate the MIPS adjustment on a sliding scale based on individual provider performance.

Using a separate adjustment code for the MIPS exceptional performance adjustment may prove more complicated and difficult since two adjustment transactions would be needed. A single adjustment code could be used for the MIPS adjustment and analysis could be based on a calculation. For example, on MIPS adjustment code could be used, but the total could be divided into the base and outstanding components for analysis. The practice/HCO may want to evaluate the return on investment between costs associated with earning the highest score versus the base score.

Policy and Setup Issues

The practice/HCO selects quality measures and clinical improvement activities that the organization will monitor and use for MIPS scoring.

- For practices that are a single area of medicine, a common set of both quality measures and clinical improvement activities should be considered.
- For multi-specialty practices, all doctors in the same area of medicine should use the same quality measures relevant to their area of medicine. However, the practice/HCO should use the same clinical improvement activities if possible. For example, some clinical improvement activities

are more appropriate for a primary care practice. Practices/HCOs that provide primary care and specialty services may need to use different clinical improvement activities for each provider type.

Practices/HCOs may choose to use more than the required minimum quality and clinical improvement activities to improve management and performance.

> *ALERT*: Practices/HCOs should refer to the capabilities of the CEHRT in choosing their quality and clinical improvement options. CEHRTs are not required to support all measures and activities. Additionally, CEHRTs are not necessarily efficient in how scores are compiled. For example, some measures are automatically calculated from clinical activities while others may require the user to check a box that the activity was completed.

Using the same quality measures and clinical improvement activities optimizes operations and simplifies management and monitoring performance across the organization.

Allocation of the MIPS adjustment for physician compensation will be a challenge for practices/HCO reporting as a group. The practice/HCO has options:

- Credit all physicians equally. If the practice/HCO received a single score, all providers could be assigned the same credit for calculating performance and/or compensation.
- Internally score each provider under MIPS. The practice/HCO could allocate the Medicare adjustment on a weighted basis to each provider based on the internal performance of each provider. Fortunately, CEHRTs can produce MIPS reports by provider to support an internal scoring process. That way, the practice/HCO can track MIPS performance with the "out of the box" CEHRT capabilities.
- Allocate the MIPS adjustment to offset practice expenses. The practice/HCO could allocate the new MIPS adjustment to lower the expenses and allocate revenue to providers based on the Medicare reimbursement amount.

> *ALERT*: Regardless of the allocation method, the practice/HCO still faces a difficult allocation of expenses decision.

For example, expenses could be allocated on usage, equally to all providers, or on a weighted basis.

Allocation of the MIPS adjustment for each qualified provider separately scored will pose several challenges. The practice needs to balance the general tactic to credit generated revenue with allocating additional MIPS costs to the providers who benefit from those investments. For example, a provider who did not participate in MIPS and did not take advantage of the changes to support MIPS may question an allocation of the MIPS-related costs to their compensation formula.

> *TIP:* Practices/HCOs should consider requiring all providers to manage and serve patients under the same standards and protocols. In that way, the CEHRT is used consistently to protect the integrity of the patient record. As important, consistent patient service procedures and strategies will improve management and service. For example, providers should not be able to opt out of a clinical call center used to support 24/7 clinical services under the clinical improvement activities or not use RPM systems for Advancing Care Information.

Enrollment

MIPS scores are awarded based on activities with patients seen during the MIPS performance period such as 2017 for 2019 adjustments. The actual adjustments are made to Medicare charges.

Patient Service Issues

The Advancing Care Information MIPS component is based on patient engagement items, including making patient information available electronically, sending a secure message to a patient, providing electronic patient education, and having patients access their information. The ACI scores are calculated from the number of unique patients seen by the provider during the performance period. The basic requirement for providing patients or their representatives access to patient medical records impacts your ability to meet the other ACI requirements. For example, if patients are not signed up for access, then you will not be able to send them a secure message in most CEHRTs.

TIP: To maximize the ACI score, the practice/HCO must enroll as many patients (or their representatives) as possible to access the patient information, typically through a patient portal. This activity should be pushed as soon as possible due to challenges of getting patients to register for patient portal access.

As a practical matter, the use of the patient portal should be offered to better serve patients than what is possible through other means. For example, the patient portal should offer quick access to the important information patients need such as their current treatment plan, patient education, secure messages, next appointment, and current prescriptions. Portals that allow access to large amounts of information may not be helpful or focus the patient on what is important and relevant.

The patient education content should be based on what is available and recommended. For example, the practice/HCO may develop specific materials on treatment strategies and protocols relevant to covered services. Similarly, Medicare Advantage services may be specified in the patient education materials about treatment options and strategies.

PMS Issues

MIPS adjustments pose a serious challenge. The traditional FFS-based PMS maintains a fee schedule for the payer and an expected payment from the payer for each service/CPT® code. In many cases, the fee and payment schedules can be specific to a payer or shared among many payers.

CAUTION—The practice/HCO should also verify how the Electronic Remittance Advice from Medicare will be posted. The posting strategy may have an impact on how you set up your reporting and physician compensation model.

Some practices may bill their standard fee while others bill the Medicare approved fee for each Medicare charge. The key question is how the MIPS-adjusted Medicare payment should be posted. For example, the practice/HCO may bill Medicare $100 and receive the adjusted payment of $96–$122 in 2019.

Depending on the operation of the PMS, the expected payment amount could exceed the billed Medicare amount. The expected payment is used to verify incoming remittances.

If the practice/HCO has submitted information for each provider separately, then the MIPS adjustment may vary by provider. For example, one provider may have a -4% adjustment while another doctor may have a +14% adjustment. To verify the Medicare adjusted reimbursement, a separate expected payment schedule should be created for each provider.

If the practice/HCO receives a group score, then the expected Medicare payment should be adjusted by the percentage assigned to the group.

> *TIP*: The actual Medicare payment could vary by a few cents from the PMS-calculated expected amount. The practice should update the expected payment to the Medicare adjusted payment for minor calculation discrepancies.

For providers or groups that have a negative adjustment, consider establishing a separate Medicare adjustment code for the write-off. The MIPS adjustment is not a contractual write-off, but rather a loss based on the decision of the practice/HCO or provider. Such a forfeiture should be separately tracked from a contractual write-off. Otherwise, contractual write-offs would be overstated and the penalties (or forfeited income) would be unknown.

> *CAUTION*: Not all PMSs can manage expected payments in excess of the billed amount.

> *ALERT*: Some PMS strategies produce an excessive number of transactions. For example, a payment could result in an open item-level payment transaction to the charge as well as a transaction for the MIPS adjustment. As important, analytical reports and physician compensation will be impacted by how the MIPS adjustment is tracked and accounted for.

CEHRT Issues

CEHRTs support meeting and tracking MIPS requirements. The practice/HCO needs to perform the setup and training needed to use the CEHRT to succeed with MIPS. Quality measures and clinical improvement activities may require CEHRT setup changes as well as training on how to use the CEHRT to properly support and record the standards. For example, a patient contact from outside the office may have to be documented with a specific form or charge code.

MIPS scores determine whether the provider or group gets a positive or negative incentive. The ACI component of MIPS is supported by CEHRTs as follows:

- CEHRTs and their patient portals have patient engagement components to meet ACI requirements.
- Provider networking measures are built into CEHRT products.
- CEHRTs have tools to monitor quality measures and clinical improvement activities.
- CEHRTs have reporting tools for supported quality measures and clinical improvement activities.

> *ALERT:* MIPS includes a measure that requires a HIPAA Security Risk Assessment to ensure that protected health information is covered by physical, technical, and administrative safeguards. Practices/HCOs need to verify HIPAA Security (and Privacy) compliance on a periodic basis.

The CEHRT fulfills the provider networking aspects of ACI. Sending and receiving a summary of care record for a referral and reconciling patient drug, allergy and problem information are all accommodated through the CEHRT.

> *TIP:* In support of patient information reconciliation as well as collecting initial patient clinical information, many patient portals support input forms to collect health history and/or history of present illness information.

> *TIP:* Continual monitoring of activities (Chapter 13) and MIPS measures should be considered to ensure earning a positive adjustment.

Reporting Issues

A CEHRT has reporting and management tools to monitor MIPS requirements. Due to the impact that MIPS has on provider payments, practices/

HCOs should monitor provider MIPS standards on a periodic basis. As important, provider MIPS scores should be monitored to address any problems and ensure a competitive score to earn the organization's fair share of the MIPS adjustment. For example, the practice may track the MIPS score by provider monthly to help providers score well personally if the providers are individually scored. If the practice/HCO is scored as a group, the individual providers should be monitored monthly to assure that the group attains their MIPS target.

> *TIP:* If a provider is not meeting the MIPS score target, consider increasing score monitoring to weekly.

MIPS CHECKLIST
General Readiness

☐ Select group or individual MIPS scoring.
☐ Select quality measures and clinical improvement activities. Attempt to use the same selections where possible.
☐ Determine how adjustment will be credited to physician compensation and production.
☐ Verify that appropriate patient education materials are available for electronic access by patients.

Implementation Items

☐ Verify how the CEHRT tracks the selected quality measures and clinical improvement activities as well as the ACI measures. Train staff and providers on the scoring requirements.
☐ Select and deploy information collection from patients outside of the office using such tools as smartphone apps or remote devices.
☐ Enroll as many patients or their representatives as possible in the patient portal.

Operational Items

☐ Verify publishing patient information to the patient portal on a timely basis.
☐ Monitor MIPS measures monthly by provider and for the group.
☐ Verify MIPS score with practice/HCO information.
☐ Monitor posting of Electronic Remittance Advice and posting of checks to support analysis and physician compensation.

CHAPTER 8

Performance and Quality Incentives

Much like the MIPS covered in Chapter 7, other payers, and ACOs may tie incentive payments to performance measures. Performance and quality incentives may directly or indirectly affect revenue. For example,

- Preferred Fee Schedules—As a condition to qualify for a preferred fee schedule, the practice/HCO may have to maintain specific performance levels.
- Incentives with a Reduced-Fee Schedule—The payer may offer a reduced-fee schedule with the possibility of earning even more money through performance-based incentives.
- Additional Incentives—Additional incentives may be offered to incentivize practices/HCOs to improve patient services and make good use of FFS reimbursements.

In any case, the practice/HCO must meet certain standards and metrics that may be based on clinical and operational performance as well as patient surveys by the payer.

The practice/HCO could have a variety of performance and quality standards spanning various plans as well as unique standards for a non-FFS arrangement. Incentives may be based on a variety of factors, from patient outreach to efficiency in operations and patient outcomes. For example, an industrial medicine operation may have a performance contract addressing days to return to work and the return-to-work status of employees.

Management Accounting

Performance and quality payments are paid on a monthly, quarterly, or even annual basis. The payment may be determined easily from quality and performance calculations that can be completed by the practice or determined by the plan based on a variety of factors and competitive standing. For example, the plan administrator may graduate payments based on performance of all practices.

The practice/HCO should track the quality and performance measures on an ongoing basis through the CEHRT. In some instances, the quality and performance requirements can be met through the standard operations of the practice/HCO and in other situations, additional investments will be needed to support the plan requirements.

The following example deducts specific costs to meet the quality and/or performance requirements from the amount available for distribution.

Quality and Performance Payment	XX,XXX
Less Costs Directly Associated with the Requirements	
Tracking Unusual Requirement	X,XXX
Allocation from Call Center	XX,XXX
. . .	
Net Surplus/Deficit for Quality/Performance Incentive	XX,XXX

The surplus/deficit can be allocated to providers using a graduated scale of performance and quality measures among all providers, or allocated to the providers based on the number of patients supported in each plan.

Policy and Setup Issues

The practice/HCO should verify that the required performance and quality measures are tracked through the PMS/CEHRT. Alternatively, the requirement could be tracked through a custom report or workaround. For example, a custom report may be able to correlate the time to contact patients based on the severity of their condition.

The practice/HCO should ensure that all users are recording patient information in support of the performance and quality standards. For example, a new process may be needed to record distribution of information to the referring provider on a timely basis.

TIP: If a plan's requirements are significantly different from the accommodations of your CEHRT, you may work with the plan administrators to come up with a comparable replacement supported by your CEHRT. For example, the practice could propose using standard clinical improvement activities under MIPS.

TIP: Providers who are not performing at the necessary level can be advised on changes to improve quality and activity performance. In some cases, the practice/HCO will need to fine-tune clinical operations and patient care to more effectively meet quality and performance requirements.

Enrollment

In most cases, the plan defines the patient base covered by the performance and quality requirements. Inclusion may be based on covered patients as well as more focused qualifications based on age, sex, and even conditions.

Patient Service Issues

The practice/HCO should check that patient services are within the performance and quality parameters of the plan. For example, the practice/HCO may have a requirement to contact patients with certain diagnoses on a periodic basis.

Patient education and interactions with the clinical staff can be used to reinforce performance and quality requirements at the patient level. For example, the patient portal could include targeted information on the treatment features of the plan focused on tactics supporting the quality and performance standards. The importance of completing the prescribed antibiotic may be included in the patient materials and followed up with a secure message to the patient on their health status after completion of the antibiotic.

PMS Issues

Patients covered under the performance and quality incentives should be easily identified through a separate plan class.

Posting of the quality and performance payment should be used to calculated performance and quality measures from the PMS and CEHRT. Any issues can be discussed with the plan administrator.

CEHRT Issues

The practice/HCO may need to design workarounds to track performance and quality measures outside of the CEHRT capabilities.

Some CEHRTs allow CDS interventions to be driven at the plan level. Thereby, the performance and quality requirements may be further highlighted with the CDS feature.

The practice/HCO should monitor performance and quality measures on a periodic basis by plan. A focus on plan is needed to avoid losing plan-specific performance among a large patient base. Additionally, plan performance requirements may differ from the quality and activity measures check to track bigger plans and Medicare.

Reporting Issues

Plans that use the quality and performance options from MIPS can be tracked through standard CEHRT reports.

Non-MIPS quality and performance measures may require custom reports or creative use of existing reports and capabilities. For example, a report of patients meeting the performance requirement may be used to calculate the performance percentage. Note that practices/HCOs should maintain supporting documentation for any quality and performance reporting.

PERFORMANCE AND QUALITY INCENTIVES CHECKLIST

General Readiness

☐ Assess the proposed Performance and Quality Incentives arrangement to track performance through the CEHRT.

☐ Design allocation of revenue to incentivize providers to support quality and performance incentives.

Implementation Items

☐ Verify coding of information to properly track quality and performance requirements.

☐ Train staff on proper recording of information to maintain quality and performance information.

Operational Items

☐ Monitor group and provider performance on a periodic basis to assure meeting goals and requirements.

CHAPTER 9

Care Management

C are management payments compensate practices/HCOs for monitoring patients with a continuing problem such as diabetes, obesity, heart problems, and depression. Under care management arrangements, the practice/HCO tracks patient wellness and triggers interventions when patient health trends are deteriorating. Care management actively encourages patient adherence to treatment plans and strategies.

Many FFS patient treatment plans are time-driven. Based on the physician's reasonable clinical judgement, the patient would return to see the doctor in six months or three weeks as appropriate. The patient's situation may evolve to require a shorter or longer period between visits. Typically, the next report on the patient's condition would occur at the next visit. The patient would have to recall any significant events such as the disease episodes and severity levels since the last visit. In many cases, these reports are anecdotal and lack specifics that could provide a more accurate view of the patient's situation. Similarly, a patient encountering a problem may delay contacting the physician to see if the problem is a troublesome trend or an aberration.

Payers are investing in care management to avoid acute care episodes and more serious problems. Monitoring patient status outside of the office may avoid office visits and appropriately timed office visits may advert a hospital visit. For example, weight gain may trigger a call from a health coach to get the patient's weight under control. Similarly, patient osteoporosis pain levels may trigger a call to schedule an appointment with the doctor or adjust medications. Dermatology staff may actively follow up with a patient on whether a mole shape has changed.

Care management strategies seek to improve patient engagement and gather patient information more frequently outside of the typical office visit.

Patient engagement may be driven by a treatment plan, a general standard of care applied to all patients based on clinical information, or an incident that triggers a practice/HCO response. Frequent calls to the clinical call center, a problematic trend reported through RPM, or a practice-driven concern about treatment can trigger a care management response. Indeed, the care management arrangement may pay for new tools to mitigate the chance of a slip in patient condition that could result in a more extensive and expensive clinical event.

Technology offers a wide range of cost-effective opportunities to continuously monitor and engage patients in managing their health under a care management program. Care management activities may include phone contact, remote device monitoring, and scheduled patient engagement. For example,

- Remote patient monitoring (See Chapter 4) allows for continuous reporting of the patient to monitor trends in the patient's situation as well as trigger a timely response to problematic subjective or objective reports.
- Telemedicine allows for more frequent patient interactions on their health status and situation at less cost and more convenience. Therefore, the patient can be more closely monitored at less expense than typical home visits or clinical exams.
- A periodic phone call to a patient may check on the patient's mobility and/ or adherence to a drug plan as part of the patient's care management plan.
- Immediate patient service available from a clinical call center may avoid an unnecessary hospital visit by addressing a patient issue or initiate a more vigorous clinical response to a change in the patient's condition.
- Practices/HCOs may contact at-risk patients who miss an expected report on their condition.

Care management arrangements can differ among payers as well as the targeted patients. For example,

- Medicare has a chronic care management code (99490) for management of patients with at least two chronic conditions requiring continual monitoring for at least 12 months. The chronic care charge is for 20 minutes of staff time under proper supervision. How and where a practice/ HCO would document and track 20 minutes of services is a clinical and operational challenge.

- Some care management agreements provide a monthly payment for patients meeting clinical criteria or for serving a list of patients provided by the payer or plan. The care management strategy may include a web-enabled scale to monitor the weight of a CHF patient or use of a smartphone camera to monitor a patient wound outside of office visits. A periodic phone check with the patient may be included in the care management arrangement.
- Other care management strategies allow at-risk patients to be enrolled in a monitoring program to eliminate frequent home and office visits. For example, HIPAA Secure Skype-like interactions with a patient may be used in place of home or office visits to make more efficient use of patient and provider time.

A practice could have more than one care management program with a payer. For example, one care management program may focus on diabetic macular edema while a separate program with separate requirements may target glaucoma patients.

Management Accounting

Care management is frequently based on a global monthly payment and scope of services. The practice/HCO may have wide latitude in the specific care management activities monitored through performance metrics or more specific care responsibilities. For example, the care management agreement may state specific contact frequency and tools to be used with patients.

Frequently, care management fees are paid per patient per month. For example,

Patients Covered Under Care Management Fee	100
Times Care Management Per Patient Per Month	$250
Equals Monthly Care Management Fee for All Patients	$25,000
Less Cost Allocation from Call Center (400 calls @$15 per call)	$6,000
Less Patient Education Materials Expense	$250
Less Monthly Expenses for Care Management	
RPM Devices ($100 per patient)	$10,000
. . .	
Net Surplus/Deficit from Care Management Fee	$8,750

Care management fees could also pay for more frequent contact with patients and be supplemented by FFS-based office visits.

> *TIP:* A care management plan may include FFS payments for selected services. For example, each phone consultation with the call center could be submitted on a claim for the patient. Care management fees based on an FFS model would be added to the monthly care management revenue as a partial offset to the care management expenses for revenue analysis and calculation of a surplus or deficit. Alternatively, the costs of the FFS-based care management services could be subtracted from the care management costs.

> *ALERT:* In many cases, the care management fee may have excessive startup costs in the initial months. For example, the practice/HCO may incur expenses to initially evaluate a patient or set up RPM devices. The practice/HCO should create a budget and consider approaching the plan administrator for financial support. For example, the practice/HCO may be paid an initial fee for the first month a patient is covered by the care management plan.

Policy and Setup Issues

The practice/HCO must examine the feasibility of fulfilling each care management arrangement. Care management services may require changes to the clinical service strategies. The practice/HCO will need to evaluate the care management scope of work and services for each arrangement. For example, an RPM device may have to be added to the treatment plan of patients who meet the clinical conditions. The practice/HCO would have to support RPM reporting and ensure that proper alert triggers were defined for the general patient population as well as the individual patient.

In many practices/HCOs, the patient service line is used to manage same-day appointments and treatment urgency by clinicians and doctors. In many situations, patient service line staff are not trained or certified to provide clinical guidance. Indeed, many patient service lines act as a conduit to patients for doctors and other providers. Care management requires active monitoring of incoming messages, patient calls, and information to clinically advise and guide the patient. For example, the patient service line may require a mid-level provider to assess the patient situation and execute the appropriate care management tactic.

The physicians will need to establish clinical care standards and guidelines for the various treatment strategies and clinical activities to support the care management program. For example, the doctors may design an initial intake patient questionnaire focusing on lifestyle and disease issues for the care management arrangement as well as targeted patient education addressing treatment strategies designed for the program at each disease severity level. The practice/HCO may design a health assessment question-naire to frame periodic reports from patients through an application on their smartphone or through the patient portal.

Care management payments frequently are made monthly. In many cases, care management requires new expenditures on staff and other items to improve patient monitoring and proactively respond to patient changes. The allocation of any care management surplus may be applied to the general organization expenses that would affect each physician in equal measure or on a level-of-effort basis to each provider. For example, the care management surplus may be allocated to providers based on their clinical oversite of the clinical call center, creation and maintenance of call center standards, analysis of results, development of new strategies, and other factors.

Enrollment

Patient enrollment in the care management arrangement may be driven by the practice/HCO, another provider such as a hospital, or the payer. In any event, care management enrollment strategies may differ depend-ing on the status of the patient and the practice/HCO. For example, if the practice is responsible for monitoring a new patient, the care management protocol may require an initial patient visit and supporting education about the condition. Interestingly, some hospitals pay for care management of discharged patients to minimize payment reductions under the Medicare Hospital Readmission Reduction Program.

TIPS: Consider using the patient type field of the CEHRT to flag patients under care management plans. A separate insurer record for each care management plan may be needed to structure the billing and tracking of care management efforts.

Patient Service Issues

The first challenge for any care management arrangement is designing an efficient strategy to support care management activities. The specifics of each care management plan will differ by the arrangement with the payer as well as the specifics of the patient situation. For example,

- Some home health visits for patients may be included in the care management strategy.
- Innovative strategies may use the clinical call center (See Chapter 6), to enhance or supplement patient care. For example, telemedicine calls with nursing staff and mid-level providers may be part of the care plan in place of more frequent doctor visits or even to screen patients before going to the hospital.

In many practices, just about any patient issue or question is handled by the doctor. With care management plans, the frequency of patient contact initiated by the patient as well as initiated by the practice/HCO requires several different patient service options and resources to ensure that the patient was appropriately served on a timely basis. Empowered staff, a clinical call center, and instantaneous access to relevant patient information affords a wide array of options to serve patients and improve care.

> *ALERT:* Empowering clinical staff to provide more services to patients requires physicians to define the clinical protocols and documentation requirements as well as a monitoring mechanism for patient care and services.

PMS Issues

Payer information may be established separately for each care management arrangement. Some PMS products allow you to create multiple plans under a payer; other PMS products allow you to group payers under a grouping code. To track and manage the care management patient base separately from the FFS patients, you may need two arrangements: one for the typical FFS arrangement and a second for the care management program. A report could be created that would include both relationships to evaluate the entire payer relationship.

Tracking the value of services and managing revenue are two PMS challenges for care management. Many care management activities may not have standard CPT® codes while some care management efforts may not be billed or reported to the payer. Nonetheless, the practice/HCO should track the performance of patient services to maintain the patient record as well as the cost of such efforts to monitor performance and profitability. For example, staff may call a patient based on a message from the patient over the patient portal, or a troubling glucose reading.

Care management may include unbillable services such as monthly RPM device charges and service fees, contacting a patient, responding to a patient message and a phone call from a patient. Paying for access to an Alzheimer support website with historic pictures from the local area are an out-of-pocket cost that may be included in a global fee.

Charge codes can be used to flag patients for follow-up contact using the CDS intervention feature of the CEHRT. For example, the practice/HCO could establish a CDS intervention to contact a patient if the last contact charge code is over two weeks old.

Billing for care management services is frequently based on a charge for each patient each month. The billing staff should maintain a schedule of the expected payment dates for all care management arrangements. In some cases, the HCO/practice issues a bill; in other cases, the payer may send a check for the patients under care management. Other payers require a separate patient claim where the care management fee is submitted at the end (or beginning) of the month. With many PMS systems, you will need to work around the traditional FFS features. For example,

- If you bill the payer monthly, you would print a list of all patients coded to the care management plan. The list would be used to produce a care management claim to the payer for each patient served. When the claims are paid, the PMS system will post the payment to the open care management fee charge codes in the patient ledger.

  TIP: Do not rely on the service code report to count the covered patients. For example, some covered patients may not have been served that month. A separate report should be produced to list all patients covered by the care management plan.

- If the payer sends you a check monthly, then you would use the same report to audit the incoming payment and verify that you have been properly compensated for patients under care management. Monthly payment may be prospective or retrospective. The analysis of the payment should be matched with the services provided during the applicable payment month.

The actual posting of a global check covering all patients can be a challenge if there is no care management claim at the patient level. Possible solutions include:

- Post the payment to a dummy patient account as an adjustment that offsets the accumulated charges for the care management services provided to patients. For example, you may have posted numerous care management unbillable charges that were written off to a specific care management write-off code (such as CMADJBC) for the payer care management arrangement.
- Post the payment outside of the PMS to your accounting system as recommended by some PMS vendors. However, this strategy does not allow you to use the realization PMS reporting and analytic tools that may be more helpful in identifying cost outliers and trends within the care management patient population.

For analysis of care management activities, the practice/HCO needs to track the efforts associated with the care management plan. A service (such as CPT®) codes report would report on services under the plan. Some systems will only report on the volume by service codes. That volume information could be separately analyzed by downloading to a spreadsheet.

CEHRT Issues

Physicians need to verify that appropriate documentation tools are available and set up to address care management requirements. For example,

- Clinical standards require tools and staff activities to support care management.
- Clinical intake forms are used to qualify for the care management

arrangement or establish a health baseline related to the care management focus.

- Documentation tools accommodate activities, such as a clinical call center activity, that may be outside of the traditional office visit and resulting encounter note.
- Reporting and analytic tools can identify patients with overdue or incomplete care management orders or activities.

The CEHRT treatment plan should include care management orders based on the scope of services. For example, a health coach or disease encounter group may be part of the care management strategy.

Patients under the care management program need to be clearly identified to ensure that the appropriate treatment and patient service are included in their treatment plan. For example, the care management payer may use a special payer identifier for the care management plan. Additionally, patient-specific performance and service parameters will be needed for each patient.

> *TIP:* CDS intervention can be used to prescribe care management items for patients meeting the clinical conditions while covered under the care management arrangement. The CDS may be especially useful in situations where a care management strategy change affects patients who are already being served. For example, a new service may be available to patients above a certain weight or with an excessive number of clinical call center contacts.

Care management requirements will be included in patient-specific treatment plans.

> *TIP:* The treatment plan should include any activity that needs to be managed, triggered, or tracked. Plan items may include the initial intake, periodic reporting, telemedicine contacts, office visits, testing and procedures.

Custom reporting tools and/or patient lists with proper filters (such as plan, diagnosis, period since last phone call) should be developed to verify that patients covered under the care management plans are being properly served. These tools may address several care management issues such as:

- Verifying the last service date was within the required time frame of the care management requirements.
- Designing the proper monitoring strategy and services needed for the patients covered under the specific care management standard for the covered conditions.

Review of the activities to date may help you identify patients who are using more resources that may need some additional care strategies to improve adherence and control costs. For example, the practice/HCO may want to identify patients who require an excessive number of calls and services to determine if any changes in strategy could be used to improve the patient situation.

Note that some care management plans may allow you to bill for more difficult or needy patients who are outliers to the care management patient base.

Reporting Issues

Financial reporting will be subject to PMS/CEHRT services recording. Ideally, the practice/HCO will use non-CPT® and CPT® service codes to post services to the PMS. Consequently, PMS reporting can be used to quantify the relevant level of services by payer and patient. For financial reporting, the number of services could be reported with a cost or charge basis to value the services provided and compare services with care management revenue.

Clinical reporting and analysis will focus on verifying the services provided to the relevant patients as well as identifying patients who have not been served within the care management requirements.

The open orders represent the future services that the practice/HCO is committed to. These orders are a valuable tool that would help you determine the prospective costs over the next month. For example, a report on the scheduled services with charges or costs would help budget the care management fees for the next month.

CARE MANAGEMENT CHECKLIST

General Readiness

☐ Assess contractual requirements of care management program.

☐ Develop best practices-based care management strategy to capitalize on the clinical, operational, and patient service advantages of the practice/HCO.

☐ Verify ability to support the patient volume and care management strategies. For example, the practice/HCO may need a home health partner to supplement the telemedicine strategy.

☐ Develop plan to flag patients under care management arrangements.

☐ Design method to track care management obligations.

Implementation Items

☐ Create CEHRT documentation tools to support care management.

☐ Set up clinical call center to meet new care management requirements and patient volumes.

☐ Verify enrollment of initial patient base for care management. Schedule new patients for initial intake reviews.

☐ Establish provisioning process for care management equipment or apps.

☐ Set up non-CPT® charges to track care management services and efforts.

Operational Items

☐ Monitor care management activities daily.

☐ Verify billing and receipts with services provided by the plan.

CHAPTER 10

Shared Savings

Shared savings arrangements pay the practice/HCO a portion of savings attained through patient service and care innovations or changes. The shared savings administrator may pay money based on comparisons with previous costs, national averages, or some other cost measure.

In some cases, the shared savings measures practice performance while other situations may reward all practices based on the performance of the plan or program. For example, all practices may get 50% of the savings divided by the number of patients served by each practice/HCO. In other situations, the practice/HCO may receive a portion of the savings based on the practice/HCO's performance in various activities. For example, counseling groups may result in lower costs for patients suffering from depression. Similarly, better patient management may produce more timely patient adherence at less cost.

> *CAUTION:* Practices/HCOs are the first line of defense in a shared savings arrangement. Success at the practice/HCO level may save money throughout the healthcare system. Therefore, a shared savings arrangement should recognize the success of the practice/HCO saving money on patient care and not focus exclusively on the lower charges from your practice/HCO. For example, additional clinical assistance from the practice/HCO may avert a hospital stay or shorten recovery time in a nursing home.

Shared savings is a constant struggle to find new ways to improve patient care at less cost. In some cases, last year's accomplishments set a new benchmark for the practice/HCO and perhaps the shared savings sponsor. At the practice/HCO level, a drop in the shared savings revenue would mean less money for shared savings expenses and physician compensation. If the shared savings sponsor resets the savings benchmarks based on prior performance, the practice/HCO will need to do better in the next year just to maintain the shared savings revenue level.

> *ALERT:* The shared savings agreement should be carefully reviewed to ensure that the shared savings plan recognizes that constant attention to patient care is a continuing cost to achieve and maintain the shared savings benefit. For example, if the practice/HCO stopped efforts to reduce costs through patient counseling and coaching, the costs may bounce back to the same level prior to the shared savings-producing activities. Practice/HCO tracking of shared savings-related costs will help clarify the investment needed to maintain the shared savings results and benefits.

Supporting standards and materials may be provided by the plan administrator to guide the practice/HCO in evidence-based strategies and tactics. In other situations, the practice/HCO may be responsible for developing and implementing ideas that make better use of resources and save money. For example, some orthopedic practices have their own physical therapy group to ensure performance and allow for more frequent collaboration with the doctor during therapy.

Saving money while caring for patients requires constant monitoring of patient care strategies and activities. For example, a monthly report may be produced to analyze patient compliance with cost savings strategies and services. A daily report may be used to verify patient monitoring efforts. The practice/HCO must maintain accurate records to ensure that the performance statistics properly reflect patient service efforts. For example, patient adherence may be stymied due to patient delays and decisions. The practice would need to maintain appropriate records about its patient service efforts and produce analytical reports that reflect the status of patient care.

> *TIP:* If your practice/HCO has developed an effective way to save money, that may be an advantage in negotiations with the shared savings plan. For example, the practice/HCO may have an innovative memory program for Alzheimer patients that could be adopted by other HCOs.

The shared savings requirements and standards may affect the practice/HCO's approach. For example,

- If the shared savings administrator defines performance standards based on their own treatment strategy, then the practice/HCO will need to invest in the resources and tools needed to meet the requirements. For example, primary care practices may have to hire a nutritionist.
- If the shared savings arrangement rewards the practice/HCO for its own savings, then the practice/HCO may develop its own treatment and management strategies. For example, the practice/HCO may pay for patient subscriptions to access a web-based diet management tool.

Management Accounting

Shared savings payments are paid on a periodic basis. The payment amount may be unknown until receipt of the payment, and the calculation may be based on factors that the practice/HCO has limited control over or for which the practice does not control the activities of others. For example, the practice may refer an at-risk patient to a specialist who does not adequately coordinate with the referring group.

An example of a monthly shared savings payment follows:

Shared Savings Payment	$50,000
Less Unreimbursed Shared Savings Expenses	
Remote Patient Monitoring	$ 3,000
Allocation from Call Center	$25,000
Patient Education Materials Expense	$1,000
. . .	
Net Shared Savings for Distribution	$21,000

The payment and supporting documentation should be analyzed to determine additional changes to address problems and capitalize on successes. For example, if a working relationship with another provider is not yielding savings, the organization should follow up with the other provider on changes to improve results and savings. In another situation, a general ASC was not dealing efficiently with procedures and recovery, resulting in less-effective and more expensive follow-up care. The practice switched to an ASC that exclusively served the specialty and practice-specific procedures to improve care and cut costs.

Policy and Setup Issues

Shared savings programs may require significant efforts behind the scenes to monitor patient treatment plans. For example, uncooperative patients could have a serious impact on shared savings. For shared savings that span groups, working relationships and coordination between practices/HCOs may require additional referral management resources and tracking tools.

Based on a review of the contract, the practice/HCO must create internal tracking systems that measure contractual obligations as well as supporting policies and procedures. For example, patient feedback on care and scheduling options such as extended hours, telemedicine care, and location options may affect patient therapy compliance and frequency.

The practice/HCO must meet any contractual obligations for clinical strategies or processes to treat and/or manage patient care. For example, the surgery scheduling process may be expanded to include counseling and therapy services to accommodate a shared savings initiative.

> *ALERT:* Shared savings investments and results do not necessarily reside within a single organization. Therefore, the practice/HCO should carefully review the implications of the arrangement to the practice. For example, post-procedure therapy may be performed by another organization even though the practice/HCO provides those services to "save money." However, the practice/HCO may provide a more innovative approach that returns the patient to work quicker which saves money for the employer.

Shared savings surpluses can be allocated to providers globally as an offset to expenses or to each provider. Since shared savings is based on global savings, the allocation methodology would not necessarily be based on the level of billing or services at the provider level. Allocation of shared savings to providers is complex. since shared savings requires operational attention and continual improvements to generate new savings. Therefore, allocation of savings to providers should be based on the savings attained by the provider for patients served, support for savings at the organization level, monitoring shared savings strategies, and/or developing new savings ideas.

The practice/HCO could allocate portions of shared savings surpluses to each aspect based on quality and performance measures using the CEHRT and custom reports targeted to the plan. For example, an appropriate treatment plan for patients with active problems could be reported as a factor to distribute a portion of the shared savings surplus.

Enrollment

Shared savings apply to all patients identified by the plan as part of the arrangement. For example, the plan may apply to all patients served through an ACO, or only patients covered by a specific large payer plan.

Patient Service Issues

Shared savings is invariably tied to patient service. If patients follow evidence-driven treatment protocols, then money may not be needed for delayed treatment or unnecessary treatment diversions. If the practice/HCO helps avoid problems, then savings can be produced at the practice level.

Where possible, the practice/HCO should track averted services. For example, if a patient participates in group physical therapy exercises over the Internet, then recovery may be quicker and less costly. As important, close monitoring of patient issues may avoid more expensive care and problems. Such monitoring can be done with comparisons of patient services before the shared savings program, comparison with comparable patient results, and even experienced differences in care. For example, a patient directed to the practice/HCO urgent care center will avoid an emergency visit to the hospital. Internally produced information may assist the practice/HCO in working with the shared savings sponsor on the organization's added value.

Practices/HCOs may take initiative under shared savings to continually fine-tune patient service to improve results and savings.

> *TIP:* The practice/HCO may coordinate with the shared savings sponsor to seek funding for initiatives that could generate savings across the entire system. For example, closely monitoring at-risk patients with additional resources may shorten hospital and nursing home stays.

PMS Issues

The practice/HCO should set up CPT® and non-CPT® codes for any services supporting the shared savings strategy. The practice/HCO may want to differentiate between unbilled services dictated by the shared savings arrangement and practice/HCO-driven strategies. For example, the shared savings agreement may require a health coach, but the practice may have added a nutrition consultation for patients.

Shared savings payments pose a challenge for most PMSs since the amount of the payment may be unknown until receipt and the payment is not associated with any claim, patient, or provider. A reasonable approach is to post the payment to an adjustment code for the shared savings plan. For analysis, the payment adjustment can be evaluated with the value of unreimbursed services.

CEHRT Issues

Whether the practice/HCO achieves savings through diligence, a proprietary care strategy, or the requirements of the non-FFS plan administrator, the CEHRT must be set up to support the strategy. For example, relevant care items should be added to the CEHRT treatment orders and the clinical checklist should support documenting information relevant to shared savings. A non-FFS ACO may determine that savings are enhanced when the handoff from the primary care provider to a specialist is monitored by the primary care provider. In other situations, a primary care provider may determine that patient sessions with a health coach and remote patient scale monitors will ensure better results at less cost.

Staff and providers should be trained on how the shared savings aspects are managed and tracked in the CEHRT.

Reporting Issues

Analysis reports are needed to monitor patient service and activities under the shared savings strategy. Additional reports are needed to quantify savings as well as report on practice/HCO activities resulting in systemic savings. For example, periodic check-ins with patients by the clinical call center may improve patient tracking and lessen patient anxiety.

The practice/HCO reports on the cost of care are needed to meet the shared savings requirements, including the monthly costs of orders in the patient's treatment plan.

SHARED SAVINGS CHECKLIST

General Readiness

☐ Analyze shared savings requirements to determine if practice/HCO has the staff, processes, and tools to support the plan.

☐ Compile historic information on comparable target patients and the cost of care.

Implementation Items

☐ Develop tactics needed to support the plan requirements. For example, the plan may require use of a patient education content, a therapy group, or a centralized clinical call center.

☐ Design internal tracking reports and procedures to monitor shared savings tactics and results.

☐ Train staff and providers on shared savings arrangements and requirements.

☐ Create shared savings supporting order sets and patient treatment tools, including clinical content.

Operational Items

☐ Monitor support for shared savings obligations.

☐ Track shared savings performance, costs, and results.

☐ Continuously monitor results to uncover additional opportunities to fine-tune patient service and cost of care.

CHAPTER 11

Episode of Care

Episode of care (EOC) arrangements, sometimes called case rates or condition specific capitation, are used mostly to address a specific patient problem. EOC payments may be made for specific treatments and care such as a hip replacement in an orthopedic practice or cataract surgery in an ophthalmic practice. EOC payments may include the facility, professional, diagnostic, and therapy costs of addressing the medical issue. EOC arrangements are widely used for home health services covering an episode of care lasting 60 days.

EOC fees may be paid at points in the patient treatment process determined by the payer. For example, the EOC fee may be paid at the completion of the procedure, but before the completion of post-procedure treatment and therapy.

Typically, the EOC covers a specific set of services such as testing, pre-procedure services, the procedure, the facility, post-procedure testing, and therapy. Services beyond the EOC specifications may be billed on an FFS basis or may be addressed by another party. For example, the payer may exclude radiology studies from the EOC requirements and require the practice/HCO to use a specific radiology group.

The actual scope of the EOC can differ from payer to payer. For example, an industrial medicine group may handle the physical therapy, but an orthopedic practice may provide all other services for a rotator cuff injury.

EOC payments free up practices to use alternatives to patient office visits for services and patient management. For example, a physical therapy plan may include HIPAA-compliant Skype-like sessions with the patient to ensure patients do their exercises daily or to check in on the range-of-motion progress during recovery.

A similar payment mechanism at a more granular level is visit payments. Visit payments pay a set fee per visit for a patient. If the patient comes in for a basic or complex problem, the same fee is paid. Like EOC, the payment covers a set of services; additional services may be billed on an FFS basis or provided by another party. Unlike EOC, the analysis of services for each visit is not going to be particularly useful, but visit payments can be analyzed across any set of days or selections. For example, the practice/HCO may analyze all services from June 16 to August 30 or focus on visit services for diabetic patients. Based on these analyses, the practice/HCO may fine-tune treatment strategies and staff utilization.

> *TIP:* Consider negotiating a visit payment agreement with options to treat patients through the clinical call center.

Management Accounting

EOC may cover services over several months. The cash flow issues are more complicated, since the actual payment trigger and receipt of payment varies. Additionally, claims submitted for the EOC payment will be for EOC-related services that are never billed to the payer. For example, the EOC claim may be associated with CPT® and non-CPT® codes that reflect the procedure, tests, and therapies provided to the patient. The actual services may be posted to track and manage services and costs.

> *CAUTION:* The charge codes entered for the actual services must be properly adjusted to avoid distorting realization reports, but still enable tracking of EOC realization. For example, assigning a cost to the case billing code as well as a cost to all unbilled charges in support of the EOC could distort PMS cost realization reports.

In some cases, FFS payments for services outside of the EOC coverage should be considered in the total realization calculation for the EOC.

EOC results can be evaluated for each case, but should also be evaluated across similar cases as well as all cases with that payer and plan. Otherwise, one outlier case may not accurately reflect the complete relationship with the payer. EOC evaluations should focus on the plan, since there may be service nuances between EOC coverage as well as differences between patient populations. For example, recovery for a sedentary patient population may be more expensive and lengthy than for a more active group of patients with the same issues.

An example of the EOC at the case level follows:

EOC Payment for Patient	XX,XXX
Less Services Provided To Date	
Diagnostic Tests	XXX
Professional Fee for Procedure	X,XXX
Facility Fee Paid for Procedure	X,XXX
Current EOC Balance	X,XXX
Less Services to be Provided in the Current Treatment Plan Orders	
Physical Therapy in Clinic	X,XXX
Remote Therapy Sessions	X,XXX
Net EOC Surplus/Deficit	XXX

The analysis includes the services that have been provided as well as the projected future services related to the case. The practice/HCO should focus on the projected surplus or deficit and not the current cash flow related to an EOC. Otherwise, the EOC analysis would overstate surpluses and understate the cost of care.

The EOC analysis may be performed at several points in the care process, at the case level or for all cases under the payer. For example, the analysis may be performed when the full treatment plan is entered, at key points in the service process, and at the end of the case. Additionally, an analysis of all current EOC cases could be created to verify that the treatment plans are meeting expectations as well as to analyze costs and results for additional care ideas. The analysis may be based on the realization of the EOC compared to standard prices, costs, or other measures.

> TIP: Clinically driven changes to the treatment plan may occur as the treatment plan proceeds.

Policy and Setup Issues

EOC arrangements produce financial benefits to the practice/HCO when the practice/HCO has a technique or strategy that will save money. For example, the practice/HCO may have a patient education program and counseling services with innovative therapy over the Internet that speeds recovery and improves results. Therefore, the physicians should strategize about improving care steps under the incentive for innovation available with an EOC. For example, payers may not pay FFS fees for remote physical therapy or counseling sessions, which may be allowed under the EOC arrangement.

EOC arrangements may be directly with the payer or with another healthcare provider. For example, a hospital may have an agreement with the practice/HCO to provide professional services under an EOC between the hospital and a payer. Of course, the practice/HCO could have a similar agreement with the hospital for facility services that the practice/HCO needs to support its own EOC with a different payer.

The EOC program should be designed to optimize the services provided to the patient and may require cooperative arrangements with other providers. For example, the practice/HCO may negotiate a service agreement with another HCO to provide services that the practice/HCO may not provide but that are included in the EOC scope. In these cases, the practice/HCO would pay the other organization directly for the services. For example, an orthopedic practice would pay the ASC directly for the patient procedure. Similarly, an optometrist may be paid a co-management fee by the ophthalmologist.

EOC payments are based on completing a key step such as the procedure, or at the end of the treatment process. Revenue is typically assigned to the providers through the charges entered for the services in support of the EOC.

When the EOC payment is received, the charges can be "paid" with the EOC payment, or offset against the write-off code used for EOC charges. If the services charge value exceeds the EOC payment, the practice would proportionally allocate the payment and analyze the process for improvements to stay within the EOC amount. If the EOC payment exceeds the value of the services, the surplus can be allocated to the supervising provider on the case, providers at the end of a quarter or year, or as an offset to expenses.

> *ALERT:* The charges representing the actual services provided are important to track the level of effort and properly

maintain the patient's medical record. However, the EOC payment may trail some charges by several months while leading other charges for services by a couple of months.

Enrollment

EOC situations are typically driven by the assignment of the patient to the practice/HCO or a treatment trigger when the patient requires services for one of the EOC treatment plans. For example, a patient may come in for consult on a problem that triggers the treatment plan and the EOC coverage for a procedure. Once a patient is under an EOC arrangement, applicable services will be covered within the EOC scope and compensated through the EOC payment.

Patient Service Issues

The focus of patient service under an EOC is adherence to the treatment plan designed by the practice/HCO to optimize care and improve results on a cost-effective basis. Practices/HCOs may be free to provide services in innovative ways within the treatment plan. For example, the practice/HCO may use online videos, Skype-like HIPAA-compliant sessions, and a case manager to support its best practices model to address the patient's problem.

> *TIP:* Practices/HCOs that seek to optimize patient care and results should track patient progress and satisfaction to further modify the treatment plan for further improvement. For example, range of motion at various points in the process as well as patient satisfaction surveys may help the practice/HCO adjust the treatment plan.

PMS Issues

The practice/HCO should track the value of services provided under each patient's EOC by posting charge codes for all services. The charge codes posted for tracking purposes may be posted and will be written off or posted at zero, depending on the PMS.

If all services are recorded in the PMS, then the analysis can be based on the actual services. Unfortunately, some organizations post only the EOC charge. In addition to billing, the lack of service codes posted to the patient account prevents the patient from being properly evaluated for quality and performance purposes. For example, a CDS intervention may not be triggered and the patient may erroneously appear on a custom report of patients who did not have post-procedure therapy.

> *TIP*: Some payers and Medicare require submission of informational claims containing relevant charge information for analysis and tracking.

CEHRT Issues

Treatment plans supporting the EOC for the non-FFS plan should be available in the CEHRT. The treatment plans may have plan-specific options as well as reflect practice/HCO-driven optimizing services. For example, the practice/HCO may use the clinical call center to verify patient home therapy activities with the plan's treatment orders.

The treatment plan for the patient should be maintained throughout the case. In that way, the practice/HCO can monitor the services to complete treatment. Interim analysis of treatment plans will allow the practice to identify problems and adjust treatment strategies to improve performance and outcome.

Reporting Issues

An analysis of patient care issues, including overdue-treatment orders and pending but unscheduled procedures, will assist staff in managing the case.

Reports on case-specific productivity and costs are needed to monitor a case as well as monitor cases by plan.

EPISODE OF CARE CHECKLIST

General Readiness

☐ Develop a best practices approach to meet the EOC service and patient management requirements, including defined relationships with other providers needed to supplement practice/HCO services.
☐ Define policy for allocation of EOC payments to services and the any surplus.

Implementation Items

☐ Set up charge codes for CPT® and non-CPT® tracking of services in addition to the EOC case charge code.

☐ Design onboarding process for new EOC cases, including treatment plan management, and patient intake.

☐ Design custom reports to manage and track the EOC cases.

Operational Items

☐ Record all charges related to the case using CPT® and non-CPT® codes.

☐ Monitor performance at the case level as well as across patients and directed to a plan.

☐ Design refinements to improve results and manage costs.

CHAPTER 12

Capitation Payments

Capitation payments are paid to practices/HCOs per patient per month and cover a set of services across a defined group of patients. For example, a primary care capitation payment may cover annual physicals, lab tests, immunizations, ambulatory care issues, and minor sickness. Services that are not covered by capitation may be paid for on an FFS basis or prohibited from being performed by the practice/HCO.

During the capitation fiasco of the 1980s and 1990s, payers paid practices/HCOs a set amount per patient per month. The practice/HCO was left figuring out how to allocate resources to meet the scope of services covered by the capitation payment. In many situations, the insurer had transferred risks to practices/HCOs that lacked the tools and procedures to manage. For example,

- No tools were available to monitor capitation arrangements and manage patient care.
- No practical alternatives for patient care were available in place of an office visit.
- Few practices changed their physician-centric patient service models. In many cases, the physician was the only one who could serve and guide patients.
- Many practices distributed the monthly capitation payments without considering additional costs associated with the capitation payments, such as known future services for patients.
- Few practices set aside a reserve to account for committed services that would be provided in future months or protect against highly unusual (and expensive) patient situations.

Success in the capitated services requires the tools, process, and management that were missing in the failure of practices/HCOs under the capitation plans of the 1980s and 1990s.

The key challenge is how to avoid the mistakes of the '80s and '90s.

Capitation plans are the ultimate opportunity to service and manage patients as efficiently as possible and optimize clinical operations. Since the capitation services are outside of FFS, lower patient care costs produce higher profits to the practice. However, higher patient costs will produce lower profits or even deficits.

The practice/HCO is constantly analyzing and reviewing patient-specific plans and general strategies to determine more cost-effective tactics and service channels. For example, if a patient can be monitored without an office visit, the practice/HCO may check in on the patient through the clinical call center. As important, patient plans are constantly reviewed to ensure the accuracy of the plan, which is critical for providing proper patient care, managing resources, and tracking future obligations. For example, patient progress may lengthen the time between office visits, or office visits may be replaced with the patient sending a picture of his or her incision to the practice/HCO on a periodic basis.

Management Accounting

Capitation payments are paid per patient per month. Some patients may receive a variety of services in the month and other patients may not be seen at all. The only way to evaluate capitation payment is across all covered patients.

Initially, the capitation payment should be analyzed with the services provided in the covered period as well as the ordered services to be provided in future periods.

> *TIP:* CDS services should be considered for patients that do not have a current treatment plan or for services missing from a patient treatment plan.

Here's an example:

Number of Patients	100
Times Per Patient Per Month Fee	$150
Capitation Plan Payment	$15,000
Less Services Provided to All Patients in Month	$10,000

Less Other Allocations	$1,000
Net Capitation Plan Surplus/Deficit for Month	$4,000
Less Future Services Costs	$8,000
Net Capitation Plan Surplus/Deficit w/ Future Orders	($4,000)

The outstanding orders for patients represent the current services commitment. Current services can be looked at for the next month or going forward for as long as necessary for the practice/HCO. Another way of analyzing the capitation plan is to match future services with the projected capitation payment.

	Next Month	Following Month
Expected Capitation Payment	$15,000	$15,000
Value of Open Order Services	$6,000	$8,000
% Encumbered (Open Services/Cap Payment)	40%	53%
Net Unencumbered Capitation Payment	$9,000	$7,000
% Unencumbered (Unencumbered Pay/ Cap Payment)	47%	60%

These analyses focus the practice/HCO on the implications of the current treatment strategy to the capitation payments. For example, the percentage encumbered may be an important metric to track future obligations.

Capitation payment analysis relies on recording services properly as well as maintaining accurate orders going forward.

Policy and Setup Issues

The practice/HCO needs to evaluate the objectives and requirements of the capitated plan to verify that the practice/HCO has the resources and strategies needed to serve patients. The requirements are a basis for designing new strategies to provide care cost effectively. For example, more mid-level providers may be hired to screen and serve patients within clinical standards set by the medical leadership. Practices/HCOs must invest time and resources to develop and implement patient service and management strategies to take advantage of the options made possible by capitation arrangements.

Using information from experiences with similar patient populations, the practice should determine the average number of services for each patient class, accounting for seasonality. For example,

- Pediatric patients would require immunizations and well-child visits while an over-65 population may require more visits and an annual EKG.
- Patient services may be lower during the summer months, but higher during flu season.

The value of the services should be used to verify the capitation rate as well as ensure financial resources to manage patients throughout the year. For example, a large summer capitation surplus should not be distributed to providers when capitation payments in the fall may generate deficits.

> *ALERT*: Practices/HCOs should be careful to manage the capitation payments throughout the year and not only in the current period.

Capitation plan surpluses can be allocated to covering future patient services as well as incentivizing providers. Provider incentives should target efficient patient services and contributions to the success of the capitation arrangement. For example, techniques to serve chronically ill patients without frequent office visits may cut down on the provider's office visit revenue, but improve the profitability of the capitation plan to the practice/HCO.

Enrollment

The capitation plan administrator assigns patients to the provider or practice.

Patient Service Issues

Like many non-FFS arrangements, the key to capitation is patient care strategies that encourage the patient to follow health recommendations and manage their care. Engagement of patients may include using the patient portal to remind patients about pending care recommendations as well as using the clinical call center to maintain contact and guide patients.

Information on the capitated services should be available to all staff to ensure that services covered under the capitated plan are provided.

A patient intake process should be used to establish the appropriate care plan for the patient. Depending on the situation, the intake process may be performed through the clinical call center or an office visit.

PMS Issues

Capitation payments are based on a defined set of services, procedures, and/or tests. Any patient service item that is not included in the capitation payment may be separately billed by the practice/HCO through a claim, or referred to another healthcare provider. Indeed, if the practice/HCO performs the excluded service that was to be performed by another healthcare organization, the practice will not get paid for the excluded service or test performed.

To meet the capitation arrangement, the terms and conditions of the capitation plan must be available in the PMS and used to manage and structure patient care. For example, procedures and treatments that are covered by the capitation plan should be available for reference and appropriately included in the treatment plan. Some CEHRTs support capitation plan requirements in their CDS feature.

For internal management and cost monitoring, the practice/HCO should post charges covered by the capitation payment to the PMS. In that way, the other PMS and CEHRT features that use the patient service codes will operate and the PMS can be used to determine the value of services provided when analyzing the capitated arrangement.

Capitation payments can be verified by tracking the census of covered patients with the patient rate.

Capitation payments can be posted to an adjustment code that is used to write off the value of covered services posted to patients.

> *TIP:* Although charges may not be billed, the charges posted can be used to track costs and patient service.

CEHRT Issues

Capitation plans may dictate what services are performed by the practice/HCO and what services are referred to other parties. For example, the CEHRT plan may require lab services to be performed by an outside lab.

Outstanding patient orders are important to allow the practice/HCO to project future responsibilities and encumbered costs for future capitation payments.

If a patient refuses services, the practice/HCO should track patient's lack of adherence to work with the capitation plan administrator on the effect of patient resistance on service levels and commitments.

Practices/HCOs need to explore the technology options that can improve patient service and control costs. For example, the practice/HCO may compare the cost of care between various facilities used to host procedures including the recovery time and cost of aftercare.

Reporting Issues

Capitation reports should include the value of the services provided over the period covered by the payment.

CAPITATION CHECKLIST

General Readiness

☐ Verify the projected costs of services included in the capitated payment to calculate the expected expenses.

☐ Analyze the capitation service requirements to determine efficiencies that could be used to improve patient service and results. Consider services that could be performed through the clinical call center and other mid-level resources.

☐ Establish clinical protocols to support capitation driven patient service innovation.

Implementation Items

☐ Set up clinical content and CDS rules to support the capitated plan.

☐ Train providers and staff on capitation innovation techniques.

Operational Items

☐ Perform intake process for new patients.

☐ Monitor patient adherence to meet capitation service goals.

☐ Track capitation expenses and realization through reports on a periodic basis.

CHAPTER 13

Monitoring Operations and Patient Information

U nder non-FFS arrangements, providers are responsible for more patient care outreach and service management. The key tool to manage and support these interactions is the CEHRT. Without the CEHRT, you cannot effectively track, measure, or manage your non-FFS arrangements.

At the end of the working day, every practice and healthcare organization performs a reconciliation of fee tickets and receipts to ensure that all charges and payments were properly posted and applied. This effort ensures the integrity and accuracy of the PMS financial records. A similar process is needed to guarantee and maintain the integrity of your CEHRT-based patient information as well as meet your non-FFS obligations.

CEHRTs include a wide array of information that requires timely handling and maintenance. Incoming patient information, internal messages on patient matters, and outstanding patient orders are a few examples of important patient issues that require timely vetting, handling, and response. CEHRTs maintain a wide range of information about what practices/HCOs do with patient issues and when they do it. These audit trails are critical tools to understand and manage practice performance as well as to prove due diligence.

Practices/HCOs need a daily clinical close process to monitor clinical activities as well as ensure that all patient information, issues, and documents were properly addressed and completed. Otherwise, the integrity of the patient medical record is undermined and patients and users lose confidence in the CEHRT-based information. Timely management of patient information is critical to meet a variety of requirements, including professional standards and some non-FFS contracts. Additionally, incomplete messages, open orders, and unsigned clinical notes may undermine the defense of a claim of medical professional liability. For example,

- Incomplete messages cluttered up a physician's inbox and the doctor missed important incoming results that were not communicated to the patient.
- An unsigned patient clinical note cannot be billed to the insurance company. Indeed, Medicare requires CEHRT-based patient encounter notes to be electronically signed within the time it takes to complete transcription.
- Open orders in the patient record included services that had been completed as well as services that had been cancelled due to a change in the patient's condition.

Each type of patient service activity moves through a clinical lifecycle. Some clinical lifecycles last a few hours; others may last years. For example, a refill request may be completed in a few hours or even in the current session while an order for annual checking of an implant may be completed within the year. Colonoscopy orders may take 10 years to complete. An alert message based on analysis of the latest spirometer reading may trigger an immediate phone call to a patient.

During an average day, each clinician may generate or respond to a hundred or more clinical events, each with its own lifecycle. The exchange and movement of these clinical events may involve several administrative and clinical personnel. However, the CEHRT's ability to support care and patient service can be undermined by not maintaining the correct status of various CEHRT items. Such lapses may be the result of a lack of training, temporary issues in the practice, or a good-faith effort to fully document a patient situation before completing the patient record.

The CEHRT audit trail is an important consideration for your clinical close strategy. CEHRTs maintain audit trails of access, viewing, editing, and other activities for each action by each user. In many cases, these audit trails are not displayed on the viewing screens, but are reportable. For example, you can get a report of every activity associated with an order or note. Timely completion of clinical items and notes ensures that the practice/HCO will not have an audit trail that may undermine clinical performance or measures. For example, a report on the time to address patient questions may be based on the audit information

The daily clinical close process will vary based on the size of the practice, operational issues, and the capabilities of the CEHRT. For example, each satellite office may handle daily note and message checking for the office, but global checking for overdue patient service orders may be handled by the main office. In some cases, separate software systems are used for the CEHRT, patient portal, and RPM. Each system would have to be separately managed and monitored. The clinical call center may monitor items throughout the day to ensure timely vetting and response. In cases where the CEHRT does not have the tools to support a daily clinical close process, the practice/HCO may need to rely on a report writer.

Framework for End of Day

The following list of clinical items and daily clinical close considerations provides a framework for the practice/HCO end-of-day process.

Exam Note Sign-off. Patient CEHRT notes require a sign-off to acknowledge completion of the patient encounter. Signing the note is essential to document physician approval of the note and plan for patient treatment as well as document the level of service. With the best of intentions, some physicians prefer to leave notes unsigned in case a subsequent event affects the analysis or plan. However, without checking each note, notes could remain unsigned long after the patient is seen. Some CEHRT systems will automatically lock the note without the doctor ever signing it. However, providers should sign their own notes within a timeframe to meet billing and documentation requirements.

> *Daily Close for Exam Notes.* The daily close process for exam notes will verify that all exam notes have been signed within 24 hours or whatever time is determined by the practice. Note that CEHRT-based exam notes must be signed within the time needed for transcription per the Medicare billing rules.

Messages. Messages from the patient portal or the phone must be tracked as the issues are forwarded to appropriate clinical staff for review and/or resolution. The responsible clinician may refer the problem to another party, talk to the patient, or send the clinical decision in a secure message to the patient. Alternatively, the provider may send instructions back to the clinical call center to follow up with the patient through the patient portal or with a phone call.

When a patient service activity is recorded, acted upon, and completed will determine whether emergent issues are addressed and coordinated with the patient. From a practice management and quality perspective, timely response to patient issues may impact quality measures, patient satisfaction, and incentive payments.

Failure to maintain appropriate status of messages could lead to cluttered inboxes that will confuse doctors and staff. For example, a "review lab results" message may remain open for results that have been reviewed. New documents may be displayed as already been reviewed. Users will waste time looking for the open tasks or, in the worst cases, stop using messages and tasks to document activities.

> *Daily Close for Messages.* The daily close process for messages will review the aging of messages by classification. For example, post-procedure questions may have to be answered in an hour while prescription refills should be addressed within the day. Special attention should be paid to secure patient portal messages from patients to ensure timely response to patient issues. For example, a patient who does not get a timely response to a secure patient portal message will call the practice and may stop using the portal.

Orders. Patient orders in the CEHRT reflect the recommendations to help the patients stay well or improve upon their current condition. Orders have due dates with a variety of implications, depending on the patient's condition, status, and/or progress. Depending on the type of order and patient situation, the practice/HCO may need to follow up with the patient within a few days or weeks of the recommended due date.

CEHRT systems accept orders for future services such as tests, procedures, and therapy. Orders may be fulfilled by a service provided by the practice or a report from a third-party provider. If the order status is not properly maintained, the display of patient orders on the patient summary screen will be incorrect and management tools to survey open orders across all patients will be distorted. Distortions of the order status or the inability to use adequately specific order statuses may confuse staff and distort performance and quality reporting. For example, a patient order may not be fulfilled due to a change in patient status or a change in the recommended clinical protocol.

Ideally, order information should be highlighted on the patient portal and reinforced by staff when the patient calls the practice. For example, a call for a refill is an opportunity to remind the patient about an overdue blood test.

> *Daily Close for Orders.* The daily close process for orders could verify that all patients seen that day have an order for the next service. Additionally, all same-day orders should be completed within a reasonable time based on the order status. For example, an in-house lab order may be completed within the day, but a lab sample sent to an outside lab would be completed within the week.

> *Weekly Order Review.* On a weekly basis, orders that were originally entered for future services should be reviewed. Open service orders may be managed by order type (e.g., annual physical, annual implant check) or by overdue aging category (e.g., A1C labs overdue by a week, x-rays overdue by a month). The clinical guidelines will determine if a reminder will be sent through a secure message or a phone call.

>> *TIP:* Depending on the weekly order review, the order status should be updated and managed to ensure accurate patient management and quality measures.

Test Results. Test results are received throughout the day from labs and diagnostic providers. In some cases, the information is loaded into the CEHRT pending review. In other cases, the practice/HCO may need to access a website to download the information. Any incoming results and observations need to be reviewed and analyzed to update the patient's treatment plan and/or contact the patient.

> *Daily Close for Test Results.* All test results should be reviewed within a timeframe determined by the practice/HCO. Different time requirements could be established based on the outcome (positive versus negative), patient condition, and type of test. For example, a positive finding should be reviewed within the session.

Incoming Referrals. Incoming referrals and patient information arriving through electronic summary of care records or a faxed referral letter require timely vetting and follow-up. Having the information available through the CEHRT is only part of the solution. The practice/HCO needs to monitor the importance of the referral as well as the responsibility of the practice/HCO under the relevant non-FFS arrangement. For example, the practice/HCO may be required to contact the patient within a week of receipt of the summary of care record or sooner as requested by the referring party.

> *ALERT:* Handling of patients new to the practice should be addressed in the relevant non-FFS or practice procedures. For example, the practice/HCO may have a standard response time based on the Patient Centered Specialty Practice requirements.

> ***Daily Close for Incoming Referrals.*** The incoming referrals should be reviewed daily to ensure that all referrals have been vetted and a patient message created for the appropriate follow-up. For example, a task may be created to call the patient within the four-day period established by the practice for new referrals.

Remote Patient Monitoring Information. Information from RPM devices such as scales must be vetted and addressed on a 24/7 basis. The initial analysis is performed by the underlying analytics engine associated with the service. If patient information is outside of acceptable tolerances set for the patient or globally by the practice/HCO, an alert message is sent to the clinical call center or designated provider. RPM information that is not addressed on a timely basis could represent a missed opportunity to address a patient's health status change and avert a more serious problem.

> ***Monitoring Remote Patient Information.*** Unlike the other forms of information, remote patient monitoring should be immediately vetted and acted on. The practice/HCO should have a mechanism to verify the response as well as appropriate entry into the CEHRT. The practice/HCO should consider reviewing all RPM patient records on a periodic basis to check on reporting frequency and trends that may not be detected by the patient or global rules. For example, a patient may frequently come close to the alert reading.

Incoming Patient Information. Patient information from patient portals, secure messages, and other sources will be an increasing important role in identifying patient service opportunities as well as adjustments to improve outcomes and control costs. The patient information must be vetted and addressed before being added to the patient's record.

> *Daily Close for Incoming Information.* The daily close process for incoming information includes checking the incoming information throughout the day for issues that must be addressed. The daily close process verifies that all issues have been properly addressed and completed.

Outgoing Patient Information to HCOs. Practices/HCOs send out a wide array of documents and information electronically to a variety of other providers. Electronic prescriptions to pharmacies, lab orders to hospitals, and summary of care records to specialists are sent daily. Outgoing electronic information is sent to a queue for transmission to the appropriate party such as a Health Information Exchange, or clearinghouse. Most CEHRTs send fax images to another program to send the fax.

> *Daily Close for Outgoing Patient Information to HCOs.* Each type of outgoing transaction queue should be checked to follow up on failed transmissions. For example, the outgoing fax queue should be checked for any failures and the outgoing electronic transaction queues should be checked for any pending or failed transmission items. Practice/HCO staff should follow up on any failed outgoing transmissions to fix the problem and resend the failed items.

Outgoing Information to Patients. Doctors and staff send out solicited and unsolicited information to patients on patient service issues of varying importance and timeliness. ACI encourages practices/HCOs to electronically engage with patients. Most CEHRT products support sending patients information through a patient portal; however, the practice/HCO needs to verify that patients have reviewed important information.

> *Daily Close for Outgoing Information to Patients.* Information that is published to the patient portal should be checked to verify that the patient reviewed information within parameters for each type of information. For example, a comment on a lab test would

be followed up on if the patient has not reviewed the information within three days through a follow-up email or phone call. On the other hand, the practice may not follow up with patients on patient education or normal clinical notes posted to the patient portal. The outgoing fax queue should be checked for failed patient documents. The practice/HCO should follow up on any patient fax failures.

Document Review. Incoming documents may be received by fax, mail, or electronic transmission. The document is scanned or loaded into the CEHRT as soon as possible. Unlike paper records, electronic images can be tracked through CEHRT image or message status. However, failing to maintain the appropriate status can lead to inaccurate documentation of patient services and even missed opportunities to review the document.

Daily Close for Document Review. The daily close process for documents consists of three aspects:

1. Verify that all documents (faxes, paper, and images) were loaded into the patient record and forwarded to the appropriate party for review.
2. Review the aging of documents awaiting review by categories. For example, a stat order should be reviewed within an hour of receipt, and an order form placed by the practice should be reviewed within the day.
3. Ensure that the relevant information was posted for patient access within 48 hours and follow-up requirements such as changing a treatment plan, scheduling a patient for an appointment, and/or referring the patient to another provider was completed.

Unfilled Clinical Decision Support Interventions. Skipped and unfilled CDS interventions may require follow-up with patients or reclassification of the patient to stop triggering the CDS intervention. In some cases, the practice/HCO may need to refine the CDS intervention, depending on more granular handling of patient problems. For example, the practice may establish different CDS triggers for treatment naïve patients.

Daily Close for Unfilled Clinical Decision Support Interventions. Practices/HCOs may want to verify the reason for unfilled CDS interventions to avoid continuing notifications that are no longer relevant and may be misleading. The staff should address the patient record to document the intervention issue and/or change the status of the patient to avoid irrelevant warnings. For example, a patient may have changed treatment strategies but the patient diagnosis code is still triggering the CDS intervention.

Whether the CEHRT includes explicit tools or requires a workaround to monitor patient service items, the practice/HCO must monitor performance and ensure that all patient issues are addressed on a timely basis. The ability to monitor and manage response to patient service issues through the daily clinical close process is contingent on the consistent use of the CEHRT by staff and providers as well as the timely recording of all activities in the CEHRT.

The daily clinical close process should be based on a set of standards established by the medical leadership over clinical activities and tolerances for response or completion. For example, doctors may have to sign exam notes before the end of the day. As important, the daily clinical close process requires the support of medical leadership and management to ensure that problems are addressed.

The actual daily clinical close process will depend on the features and functions of the CEHRT. Options include:

- **Worklists**: Some CEHRTs allow you to set up selection criteria by various types of information and produce worklists of selected orders, notes, messages, and other selected documents. The worklist can be used to access the selected items and proceed to view the item and perform various tasks. For example, you could work the message, assign the message to someone else, increase the priority of the message, and/or send a message about the item to the appropriate parties.
- **Screen Viewing**: In the event the CEHRT does not have worklist tools, you may need to view the work screen of each user and/or provider to identify items that do not meet the daily close requirements. For example, you may look at the doctor's list of incoming messages for overdue messages and the schedule for unsigned appointment notes.
- **Reports**: Systems without worklist tools and screen-viewing options may have a report writer that could be programmed for a report for each

type of information and aging category that is needed. For example, a custom report could be created to list orders for radiology studies that have a due date more than two weeks old. The report would be reviewed and overdue items followed up.

Recovery from failure to maintain the various life cycles of your CEHRT could be an expensive and time-consuming effort. More seriously, the collateral problems could be felt for many months or years thereafter. For example, orders that have not been maintained will create false overdue order messages or CDS interventions.

A daily clinical close process will allow you to monitor and maintain your patient service records and documentation to avoid distorting your patient records and document your due diligence in patient service and meeting non-FFS care requirements. Your efforts will ensure that you have the patient service management information needed to serve patients, monitor performance and maximize revenues.

CLINICAL DAILY CLOSE CHECKLIST

Exam Note Sign-off

- ☐ Establish standard to meet care and billing requirements.
- ☐ Review all appointments daily to verify exam notes were signed on a timely basis.
- ☐ Verify that supervising provider co-signs mid-level orders and notes as necessary.

Messages

- ☐ Define strategy to specify and track message handling and resolution. Message standards may be defined by message type (e.g., refills, follow-up question).
- ☐ Consistently classify messages to ensure the message categories can be properly tracked. Message classes will vary by the type of practice and services as well as the capabilities of the CEHRT. Examples of message classes include:
  - – Refill Requests
  - – Current Patient Questions

- Receipt of Lab Results
- Notification of Test Results
- Referral Request
- Surgery Scheduling
- Miscellaneous Inquiry

Orders

☐ Verify that all patients seen today had a current care plan for the next visit or treatment plan unless the patient is being released from care (i.e., sent back to the primary care provider). Primary care practices and chronic condition specialists will have continuing care issues for most patients.

> *ALERT:* CDS interventions are a backstop strategy to treatment orders.

☐ Check status and follow-up on overdue orders.

Test Results

☐ Verify that positive test results are reviewed within the timeframe established by the practice/HCO.

Incoming Referrals

☐ For specialists, verify incoming Summary of Care triggers timely contact with patient and follow-up with doctor.

Remote Patient Monitoring Information

☐ Verify that all alerts were reviewed and responded to on a timely basis.
☐ Verify that patients who were expected to report through RPM did submit information as well as following up with patients who were expected to report but didn't.

Incoming Patient Information

☐ Review incoming patient information on a timely basis to ensure that patient issues are addressed and responded to:
- Submission of information for an appointment such as HPI and medical history
- Secure messages from a patient

– Other information from a patient

☐ Produce an aging report of incoming information to identify pending follow up with patients that have not been completed.

Outgoing Patient Information to HCOs

☐ Verify that all outgoing electronic and fax queues do not have failed transmissions.

☐ Verify outgoing information to patients was sent.

☐ Verify that patients have seen critical information posted to the patient portal. Follow up with patients who have not reviewed important information.

Document Review

☐ Verify that all incoming documents have been added to the CEHRT-based patient record.

☐ Review aged incoming documents to review and act on the document within 48 hours.

Unfilled Clinical Decision Support Interventions

☐ Review overdue CDS interventions for patients seen today. If appropriate, update the patient record to eliminate inappropriate CDS interventions.

CHAPTER 14

Go-Forward Strategy

C apitalizing on the transition to the non-FFS based payment and patient service models is challenging for any practice or healthcare organization. The evolving non-FFS environment will grow while the FFS-based revenue streams will contract or be tied to non-FFS incentives in some fashion. From reduced FFS schedules with a companion set of performance requirements to capitation and EOC payments that provide incentives to improve efficiency, practices/HCOs will be facing more financial success tied to increasing responsibility for managing patients.

The bottom line is to be prepared for a variety of strategies and tactics included in non-FFS agreements. Understanding that non-FFS arrangements present serious operational and clinical challenges but also financial rewards is the first step to success. The practice/HCO needs to:

Build a non-FFS Practice/HCO. Non-FFS arrangements require an organization that is focused on collaborating with patients and other providers as well as being fully engaged in helping patients take care of themselves. Right, wrong, or indifferent, helping patients stay aware of what is needed to stay well or get better is a responsibility delegated to your organization by many non-FFS strategies. If you help the patient succeed, you may earn an incentive, cut costs on an EOC, or have a lower cost of care under a capitation model.

Certain parts of success have been established and other parts are up to you. For example, patient access to their medical data is an ACI measure, but a clinical call center and use of mid-level providers to quickly respond to changes in patient status is an organizational decision.

Negotiate to Your Strengths. Practices/HCOs need to consider what they can do to accommodate a non-FFS arrangement and what is not possible.

To succeed, the various performance, quality, and patient service requirements must be accommodated by the practice/HCO. Otherwise, the practice/HCO could be facing a non-trivial risk of loss. For example, failing to meet performance measures since your CEHRT doesn't accommodate the requirements or the inability to track outstanding services on almost any non-FFS arrangement may undermine the operation, risk patient safety, and present serious financial loses.

Refine Clinical Strategies and Tactics. Practices/HCOs need to continually rethink patient service and care. They need to pay more attention to consistency among providers and staff as well as build a cooperative relationship with patients. To succeed in a more complicated payer environment, practices/HCOs must more seriously consider all healthcare customers they serve. Your organization needs symbiotic relationships with patients, payers, and other healthcare providers to ensure that all participants are helping each other achieve success.

Train Providers and Staff. Training staff and providers is essential to ensure that the integrity of patient records is maintained and that proper records are kept to support tracking and analysis of patient care and non-FFS requirements. For example, new treatment strategies to address an innovative therapy may require new documentation tools as well as specific ordering information. Such a process may require the collaboration of the provider, referral manager, and therapy department.

Evaluate Results. Practices/HCO must constantly analyze operations and results to seek out new patient service tactics as well as adjustments to procedures to improve productivity and results. As important, practices/HCOs must constantly monitor the various quality measures and clinical improvement activities that payers and plans will use to decide whether they have earned the incentives for outstanding patient care and cost controls. More importantly, practices/HCOs need to monitor themselves throughout the year to ensure that they are on target for patient care and incentives.

Practices and healthcare organizations are at the front line of the industry effort to operate more efficiently and effectively. A wide array of measures and standards are providing a new framework that is based on non-FFS business models. Successful migration of your organization to accommodate these arrangements while being more creative and proactive in your clinical operations will help providers and staff succeed in new business models while improving patient services and results.

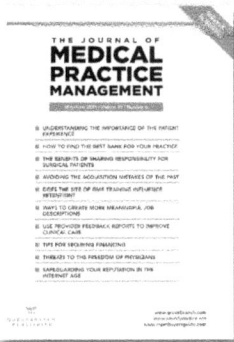